BRIDGET HAI

FINE
(Not Fine)

Perspectives and Experiences
of Postnatal Depression

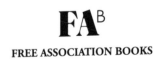

FA^B

FREE ASSOCIATION BOOKS

First published in 2015 by
Free Publishing Limited

Copyright © 2015 Free Publishing Limited

A CIP Catalogue of this book is available from
the British Library

ISBN: 978-1-8534322-0-0

Front cover images sourced through royalty free photo libraries:
© TomFullum | istockphoto.com, © Nuarevik | istockphoto.com,
© Photomak | Dreamstime.com

Cover design and typeset by
www.chandlerbookdesign.co.uk

Printed in Great Britain by
TJ International, Padstow, Cornwall

Dedication

This book is for all the mothers, starting with my own.

And for all the fathers, especially my own – in the words of my brother - "amazing, but dead, dad".

And for the father of my own babies, husband, and erstwhile colleague, Ben.

And for all the babies, starting with my own.

CONTENTS

Introduction

Most mothers, and indeed parents, describe the experience of having a child as magical. In fact in the days after my first baby was born, a friend even told me, "It's a magical time, those first few days." I remember repeating this to my husband wryly: we shook our heads and braced ourselves for another day.

Of course the birth, and the first few hours of knowing we'd brought our baby into the world were emotional, and very happy, filled with phone calls to the grandparents and messages to friends. But, for reasons which may have everything or nothing to do with the difficult circumstances which surrounded the birth, the first week of my son's life was the worst of mine. The following weeks were no better.

Initially, everyone diagnosed baby blues. Relentless exhaustion, tears, lack of bonding – many mothers tell that tale. There's no doubt that for many, parenthood is a deeply shocking experience, something sophisticated educations and focused career paths do nothing to prepare us for. But I knew there was something else: I'd experienced depression once before, I recognised its dread sensation with despair.

I was in a lost place, sick at the thought of life itself. The feeling grew worse. Perhaps knowing so soon was the one thing which mitigated the experience for us: early recognition forced family and, importantly, doctors, to admit it was a clear case of post-natal depression, and to act accordingly. The three things which got me through were medication, counselling, and infinite support from family and friends.

Now, I look at my little boy, I feel all the love I was told I would. But I also feel grief that the early weeks and months of his little life were overcast, and sometimes I wonder if I can make up the deficit of care to him, even if it takes a lifetime. I do feel forearmed if there is a next time. I know it could strike again, but this time I'll be fighting from the start.

I wrote this short note about my experience of PND before I became pregnant with my second child, after whose birth I would succumb to PND again, though I did not know it at the time of writing. During that second pregnancy I began to reflect further on that first experience of PND, to seek a way to understand it, and to try to work out if I could prevent it happening again. Although I was unsuccessful in pre-empting a second bout of PND, it was therapeutic looking back at how far I had come, and it opened up conversations with friends and strangers alike on the experience. After my second son was born, and I was sufficiently recovered, I began to collect these stories, to record them alongside my own. This book is therefore both my own PND journal, and a series of windows into other people's struggles. I've also been very fortunate to meet with some incredibly skilled and experienced perinatal professionals along the way, who have each given their own insights into the mental health issues mothers – and fathers – can face.

1

Pregnant with #2, reflecting on #1

First pregnancies are unique. Everything is new, everyone's pregnancy and birth stories are fascinating, the magazines and books have an appeal that is completely lost in subsequent pregnancies, or so I found as I planned for my second child. The trend, certainly in women of my age and background, is to immerse and educate ourselves, as if the theory will necessarily mean the practice is, if not easy, then straightforward and semi-predictable.

My generation has been raised that way. And coming to motherhood after a decade in work filled with logical thought, rational decisions and strategy planning, made me think that learning and preparation would lead to success and achievement. Those are the terms I came to motherhood on. Little wonder that I would be disappointed. Hindsight, but more forcefully, coming to know my first child, taught me that the first thing pregnant women need to know is there are no rules for babies. There is no planning. Prepare yourself for the unpredictable, the uncontrollable, put aside your regimented life, lower your expectations and the standards you set yourself.

One of the many things I learned in my copious pregnancy reading, and which I conscientiously warned my husband about, was post-natal depression. The statistics were worrying: some books had it at as many as one in four women succumbing to what had become less of a stigmatised affliction, more of a common experience. I knew enough to recognise that the dramatised version in which women experience hallucinations or seek to harm their children does not represent the majority of PND cases, psychosis is something quite different from depression. How equipped I was, how prepared when I solemnly told my husband that, given some past brushes with depression, I was quite possibly a candidate. What I hadn't realised was that while I'll never know if previous depression affected my chances of falling into the PND bracket, being someone who is not laid-back, who likes control, who doesn't for instance like the feeling of losing something or not knowing when something will happen, those factors would play far more of a role.

The causes of PND intrigue me. I've heard arguments that it is purely hormonal; extraneous circumstances are irrelevant. Yet my own traumatic experience of serious illness in pregnancy and immediately after the birth, of a difficult hospital stay and many contributing factors along these lines belies this. During my second pregnancy I took part in a research study being carried out by the local mental health trust. The study was examining the correlation between stress in pregnancy and subsequent post-natal depression, and in mother/baby relations. Second time around, I felt I was trying to do everything differently. Nobody who has experienced PND wants to get it again. Yet I knew women who had had PND twice or more, and I would flit between not wanting to become a self-fulfilling prophecy, and not wanting to be unprepared.

People often warn that new motherhood is lonely. Not so in a busy city, particularly when your immediate environs are known for a disproportionately high number of young families. But depression makes new motherhood lonely. It cut me off from my immediate peers, because I felt they couldn't possibly understand. And I felt unbearably jealous of their happiness. Of their *normality*. I turned to old friends, both with and without children, and to family. Sharing details of my condition was completely sporadic and irrational. Sometimes I would blurt it out to someone I didn't see often, knowing they were sensitive enough not to judge me. Yet there are friends I've known for years who know nothing of any of this. It's no reflection on them. It's probably a random instinct, to be seen at least by some people as just an ordinary new mum. I still find it hard listening to people chat away about the opportunities for socialising and making new friends that having a baby can bring: the little friendship groups, the mother and baby events. I barely left the house for the first five weeks because my anxiety over what would happen if the baby suddenly needed a feed, a nappy change, to scream (or that I would), was completely paralysing. The afternoon my GP prescribed my anti-depressants, she told me: "These are not happy pills. But they should give you the extra boost you need to get out and do things – and that in turn will help make you feel better." Very true, and thankfully I heeded her advice. But she followed this up with "Today for instance – it's such a lovely afternoon, you should be out in the park with the pram." I looked at her as if she was the one with the mental health problem. She may as well have said I could take the baby to the moon. I felt as though something so simple, so easy for other people, would never be in my grasp. It had taken all my courage, my energy and resolution just to get to the surgery that day with my baby. Most appointments in those early weeks I'd had to summon my mum or my husband to come with me. Handling a newborn baby seemed to me the most impossible job I had ever undertaken.

2

The beginning

I try to trace events back to the beginning, but I don't know where that really is. Is it the part where I found it impossible to keep work stress in perspective? Or where I developed pre-eclampsia late on in the pregnancy, did that pre-ordain the outcome? The diagnosis certainly necessitated a two night stay in hospital which for some reason drove me to near distraction and despair – a nasty forewarning of what seven nights post birth would do to me, with the added element of no sleep and a new dependent I didn't know what to do with. A seemingly straightforward birth that seemed to take a wrong turn, a too-small baby needing to be yanked out, a disastrous attempt to breastfeed, with all the well-documented feelings of fear and failure that can go with that. Certainly the pressure was on throughout the pregnancy – chiefly from myself – and that continued afterwards – still from myself, but also from midwives and paediatricians, often at odds with each other. Feed this small jaundiced baby, it doesn't matter what with. Feed this baby only with donated breast milk and prioritise the breast-feeding. Don't breastfeed for now, the main objective is to get fluid into him. Worse than this was a lack of understanding. "What can I feed my baby? I've run out of (donor) milk, I've not managed to breastfeed him yet," I pleaded with a night duty midwife. "I can't help you," came the blunt reply. In fact, behind her was a cupboard of formula, which for some reason neither of us thought to look to for our solution. The desperation as I cradled my tiny underweight baby. Don't carry your baby around, it's against health and safety. Don't put your baby down, you need to establish the bond and breast-feeding. Take your baby up to another floor for antibiotics he doesn't even definitely need, though your legs have only just started working, and as you stand up a mass of blood lands on the floor.

For people used to knowing what was going on, to being in control, seven days in a post-natal ward in a busy London hospital was a nightmare. Add to this the nature of the birth, the fact the baby would not sleep except on me and I was too terrified to fall asleep this way, sheer exhaustion set in after two days. Pre-eclampsia worsened – flashing lights from soon after the birth, and blinding headaches are my memories of those first 24 hours many recall as a blur of joy. You just need fresh air. You are probably just tired. The obstetrician was paged 24 hours ago. We're doing all we can.

Alongside all of this, the pain of being apart from my husband, at the time I needed him most. We had not spent so many nights apart since early in the relationship. On a practical level, I needed him to share the burden of wakefulness with me. I know now that tiredness plays a major role in depression. By the first night I was almost constantly in tears, and very afraid. "You can't afford to cry," a midwife chastised me as I struggled to get my baby to feed from me. Later I would recall those words, like a wound, a wound I picked over and used as a trigger for self-pity.

My husband describes our outlook during that week of hell as "siege mentality". Actually this became almost literally true when London was shut down by a snowstorm. We refused all visitors. Both sides of the family were desperate to meet our son, but we felt unable to cope with that, coupled as it felt to a mood of celebration. We weren't ready to celebrate; we were in a constant round of tests, feeds, observations, consultations. Nothing was ok. For a very long time after I had Joe, really until recently, I found it difficult looking at those post birth pictures people share. Everyone looks happy and unphased by the new baby, even when they're still in hospital. Of course, now I know better and can see that what isn't being shared is just as significant.

Today, I'd like to enter that ward unseen, visit the mothers there and tell them a few things. Gently take the baby so they can sleep. Tell them what to do if the baby isn't feeding. Tell them to fight their corner or get their husbands to do it for them. Tell them where the laundry cupboard is to change the bloodied sheets, which so many, including myself, end up having to lie on for too long, until a helpful friend or partner changes them for us. Tell them they are doing so well, just to have delivered their baby, let alone having started this most difficult of jobs. I want to hold their hands, even the ones who seem fine. I want to show them how to change their baby's nappy and boss the doctors around when they give conflicting advice. In truth, I'd like to go back and do that for myself too.

When I first became pregnant with my second child, I was very anxious, nervous of ending up back in the place where I felt my nightmares had begun. But, with welcome serendipity, I began to hear anecdotal evidence that much had changed. Staffing levels were improved, breast feeding help was reportedly less patchy, partners were now permitted to stay the night. This last one made me want to weep with relief. In some ways that relief was more for women having their first child: second time around I felt I might not even need my partner to stay, as by then we had an older child I was anxious should not be without one of us for too long.

This feeling of relief was not to last. The initial euphoria over a second pregnancy and relief when the early signs looked good gave way to an irritating anxiety over repeating the experience of the first birth and aftermath. My mind felt surprisingly inflexible; repeating rational thoughts and more stern exhortations (fortunate to be in this position in the first place, life is short and should be enjoyed, pregnancy will give way to manic life involving two small children so make the most of it, second birth can't be as bad as first, even second visitation of PND can surely not be so bad?) – seemed to make no difference.

Partly, I had (again) read too much. I knew that PND could strike again, particularly if you are classed as being 'pre-disposed' – though how one is classed as such, I don't know. At night, pregnant with my second child, I would lie in bed mentally arraying my artillery. Cognitive Behavioural Therapy (CBT) had been suggested by several people. Speaking to a consultant obstetrician to get the 'medical' take was another plan: was there an argument for not going down the home birth route I was planning, and hoping for, to exorcise some of the demons from my first birth. I thought about telling my midwife honestly that, despite my glib declaration that I was all better now and ready for that home birth, I was actually shit scared. On closer examination I realised that, though I had coped ok up to a point last time, this time I was afraid the first contraction would lift the lid to Pandora's box, that labour would be the worst flashback of my life – the gateway to the depression that nearly pulled me under last time. So it didn't matter when people said it would be easier, quicker, and more manageable this time. Because what if it unlocked the horror again, just by being the same set of physical launch pads? Would I be adding to this history in a few months' time?

What is surprising, and very comforting, is the level of understanding shown by women I talk to, both in person and online. Despite the occasional 'I suffered through four births without pain relief, why shouldn't you?' approach, most women are largely sympathetic, especially when they know the history. And it turns out many are in similar positions. Hypnotherapy was recommended as another strong defence, and my thinking was – what is there to lose? There is not much I find harder to cope with than loss of control, and what is more uncontrolled than a natural birth? So somehow I needed to find a way to make sure it did not undo me. Now, it felt, there was even more reason to stay sane. Not just my new baby, but my toddler son, who was going to need his mum when his world turned upside down.

3

Lines of communication

I have never been a great one for keeping in touch by phone, and find email suits me much better. I like to be prepared for communication, and this exaggerated during the early months of my first son's life. Emailing friends helped combat a feeling of isolation. It's how I told my best friends what was really happening. It's how I kept in touch with my husband during the day, just one liners about how many feeds he'd had, how I felt, whether I could make it to the shop for some milk. These probably served as a useful barometer to him of how I was feeling. Texts too were useful – how many appointments and meetings with friends did I cancel by text? I didn't want the comeback of rearranging another day, when I didn't know if another day would be the same or worse. The day I caved in and took the decision to start taking the anti-depressants I'd obtained a week or two earlier, the decision was made by text. I'd cancelled a friend coming over by text. It seemed impossible to think I could handle talking to someone I didn't know that well and not show the craziness that was going on underneath. I struggled through a feed. The thought of the next step – of changing the baby's nappy – was too much.

But I was in an inexorable cycle: feed, change nappy, it *had* to be done this way because that's what I had been told in hospital. I burst into tears. I don't know how much later it was but, by now a sodden mess on the sofa, I texted my husband, who was on his way to a meeting with a colleague and in no position to do anything, as I well knew. He suggested I call a close friend who lived nearby. I did so, but she was in a different part of London, couldn't get anywhere near me quickly. I slid into a panic, and told my husband as much. Eventually a text came from my him: "Take the pills?!", referring to the anti-depressants I had been prescribed, and had collected, but had not yet made the decision to take. So I did – that was that. My emails from around this time provide an insight to my state of mind.

March 10th

> "… just feel as though I'm making no progress at
> all, everything still feels v bleak and impossible.
> Hopefully the drugs will kick in soon. And I will
> hopefully get referred to someone who can help
> me as well. I'm just so sick of feeling like this,
> just seem to spend hours crying and feeling
> incapable, and nothing anyone says seems to
> help. I think Ben is considering taking some leave
> so he can be with me more but that is finite - and
> quite precious time - so not sure really."

I estimate I started the medication in early March 2009 (maybe six weeks after the birth of my son), so very shortly before sending this email. I may have complained it wasn't working but in fact it was fairly effective, relatively quickly.

I didn't notice at first that I was having a few not so bad days, then even the odd good day. I would notice when I had another bad day though, and say to Ben in despair, 'it's not working, I'm just the same, nothing is getting better'. And he would try to show me that I was on an upward curve, but that this didn't mean every day would be better.

I mentioned my situation to a former colleague. Her response led to part of my recovery:

"Sorry to hear things are a bit rough at the moment. I really hope they pick up soon. My sister-in-law Liz had postnatal depression after her first baby ... She found a really good psychologist to help talk through everything and I think that was the thing that helped her most. She now helps other new mums who are struggling. She is in Oz but let me know if you want her email address, I'm sure she'd be happy to chat online."

Given how much easier I find it to communicate via email, this was the perfect solution for me. I would be able to talk to someone who was connected to a friend – thus had been recommended and wasn't a random stranger – but who was only really available on email, so there need be no social niceties about arranging to meet (and then having to cancel if I threw a wobbly) or dealing with phone calls. I could choose the time it suited me to sit down and pour out my experience, and in turn to read about hers. Emailing Liz and subsequently speaking to a counsellor were crucial to my recovery. When she first got in touch, she told me her own story. It's not my place to tell her story here, but much of what she said I could have written myself. I wrote to her initially on 21 April saying:

"My doctor gave me antidepressants which seemed to take ages to work but I think must be now - definitely seems

like things are getting easier. I just wondered what your own experience was like and what you found helped to get through it?"

Whether it was because people always say the 12 week mark is like a watershed for improvement, or whether the drugs were making the difference, I do remember feeling that this stage was a turning point. In fact, in the way that when you finally get a doctor's appointment for a medical issue that's been annoying you, and then the day comes and you think actually things are fine now, when I started emailing Liz and seeing the counsellor, I almost thought maybe it wasn't that necessary - maybe I was over the worst. In fact, I have learnt that PND does not follow a straight road. The cliché of two steps forward, one step back, is probably inverted for PND. Thankfully I didn't come off the medication once I started feeling better – a mistake which some do make. And thankfully, I did not decide I could do without talking to Liz and my counsellor. Speaking to them strengthened me, without question.

25 April – email to Liz

"Once we got back from hospital though we had that 'reality' hit a lot of people talk about and it was just a nightmare for the next five weeks or so. Ben went back to work after a week and I've never felt so low. Poor him - he used to get these desperate emails and texts from me, sent during hours of sobbing. I had that thing of just wanting to sleep - it wasn't exactly that I was suicidal, just that I wanted it all to go away. I felt like my life was just this endless round of feeding/changing/washing clothes stretching ahead of me, with no vestiges of my old life. I missed my time alone with Ben and

I even missed work! I also developed all these neuroses. I was so anxious about all the logistics involved with bottle-feeding; I'd spend hours on the net researching different ways of sterilising bottles on holiday etc. I was constantly afraid of going out, even just to see the doctor, as I was petrified of how to cope out and about with him. Already I can look back and see how out of perspective it all was, but it was very real at the time. It was ironic as when I did get out, though it was exhausting, I felt so much better. I did go on anti-depressants after a while, and though they took their time they are now working (I think - probably a combination of factors). I also was very open - I told everyone! I thought it was really important to break down some of the taboos surrounding depression and in particular post-natal depression. I'm amazed actually how common it is. My GP referred me to a counsellor which is quite helpful though I think in the period where I was at my worst, I should have had more specialist help.

It's funny - Ben said the same thing to me that your mum said to you, that I WAS doing it, which really did help. He kept saying look he's fed, clean, healthy - you're doing fine. Which did help.

I do feel much better now and this week more than ever I'm really starting to enjoy motherhood as Joe is smiley and laughing and it's getting more fun. I still feel quite scarred by it all - the birth was quite traumatic (though I guess they all are to an extent) and those first few weeks still cast their shadow."

Something I'm finding surprising in looking through the old emails, is that whilst in a way they serve as a saddening diary, charting the course of the depression, they are often surprisingly lucid. I thought I was completely out of it some days – yet I could still converse with my husband about his work, about what there was in the freezer for tea, and about my son's routine.

When I experienced PND for a second time, it was a quite unwelcome reminder of some of those harder to reach parts of depression. Everyone understands the conscious, the extraneous, the tangible: you're stressed, you don't get much sleep, you are possibly still recovering physically and not eating properly... it is a huge lifestyle change (even second time around – on which more later). But I'd half forgotten the other side, the untouchable, unspeakable side. A friend referred to the creeping dark cloud, a very good way of putting it. It's also a disconnect, a crack that seems to open up between you and the rest of the normal, functioning world. I would liken it to the feeling you get when you're watching a programme and the sound is slightly out of sync. It shouldn't matter – it shouldn't affect your enjoyment of the show – but it does, it feels a little unreal and wrong, even though it's not entirely rational. That is how I would feel even on days when my toddler was off my hands, my baby was sleeping, I was well rested and fed – so, in other words, no peripheral concerns to distract me with anxiety – suddenly I'd be conscious of the enormous looming presence of the depression itself, squeezing all the air out of the room. JK Rowling's description of "dementors" in the Harry Potter books strike me as a perfect metaphor for depression.

4

Motherhood - the reality versus the fantasy

Recently I was revisiting my first experience of PND in conversation with a very close friend. One of the things she'd found hard, she told me, was trying to help me. "You just wouldn't talk about it, or let me help." I found it easy, as I've said already, to write about my feelings, but in conversation, in person, something stopped me. I clearly remember the only time I came close to it, when Joe was about four weeks old. I said to (the same friend) "I just don't think I'm the right person to be his mum." Several years later she told me this had been heartbreaking to hear. It's heartbreaking for me to write it. And what is more, I sometimes still feel this way.

All my life, I wanted children. I was the girl who played with dolls incessantly, to a slightly too old age if I am honest. I am going to have six children, I would say. This came down to four. Then, post marriage, to two. After my first child, it was revised to one, for some time. I thought I would be a natural. And it is meant to be natural! Were there clues? When I was given a newborn baby to hold at 24, and I panicked and refused, to the bemusement of my friend who knew about my much-proclaimed 'love of children', was that a sign? When my own goddaughter and other friends' kids didn't seem particularly keen on me, I was paranoid, but I never questioned how it would be with my own children – that seemed so obviously a given, a certainty I could rely on. My friend was great with kids, she joked she was the baby whisperer. Well that was fine – I would be my own baby's whisperer, the only one I'd really need to whisper to. How ironic that a few years later, I would be paying an inflated delivery rate on Amazon to have Secrets of the Baby Whisperer and The Contented Little Baby Book delivered next day, to assuage my growing panic that I had absolutely no idea what to do with this child of mine. I even said this to a friend of mine, with a daughter two years older than my first child. "I just don't know what to do with him." She looked puzzled. I now realise this is because he was a few weeks old. I didn't need to do anything with him. But I felt the need for structure, schedule, routine. The psychologist and writer Oliver James (How Not To F**K Them Up) would perhaps put me into the "Organised Mum" category. The interesting thing about women who have always cherished the idea of children, is that they are not necessarily the ones who end up loving motherhood. The opposite is also true.

Martha's story

Martha is 40, and had her first child in 2009. Having a baby was something she had longed for, but she found the reality of motherhood very far from her expectations:

"I was very excited to become a mother the first time round; it was something I had dreamed of for years and definitely wanted very much. The reality was in stark contrast. At times, during the first six to eight weeks, I sometimes found myself wishing I wasn't a mum. This was really hard to deal with."

In common with many women I've talked to, Martha was never formally diagnosed, but it does seem pretty likely she was suffering from PND. On paper, the external circumstances which can be perceived to affect mood went well – the birth was long, but then many first births are, and she says she feels it was "without trauma". She was under the care of very supportive community midwives, and had additional support from friends and family. Her National Childbirth Trust (NCT) group were very supportive and few subjects were off-limits during their regular meet ups. But bonding with her new baby was not immediate; in fact, she says:

"I would honestly say it took me until his first birthday to look at him and feel the 'rush of love' that other people described having had at birth."

This is where expectations can be so damaging. She remembers:

"I thought I would wake up every day and feel sheer joy to see my son."

Now, it's possible it really is like that for some people. And many more will say it's like that. But for those of us who don't feel that way, it is incredibly isolating. The strain of having a newborn, the reality of how much tending they actually do need: Martha describes the anxiety of hearing her baby snuffle, waiting for him to wake, and I well remember those tenterhooks. Living day to day like that, on top of serious sleep deprivation, clearly takes its toll. And despite saying her labour was straightforward, in hindsight Martha can see that 24 hours in labour was of course exhausting. She went without sleep for a long time before the baby was even born.

Alongside this, she found the tiredness of having a new baby overwhelming, and remembers feeling very sensitive. She didn't feel her husband was hugely supportive at first, saying "I needed him to read my mind, bring me sandwiches, huge glasses of fresh water… tell me I was doing a great job, offer to wind the baby in the middle of the night. I needed a wife, basically!" It wasn't all bleak – she talks about looking at pictures from the time, and seeing that there were clearly happy days too. But simple things, like not being able to finish a sandwich, or have a cup of tea – the baby always waking just as she started to eat – took their toll. Interestingly, PND was the one topic that was never brought up within her NCT group. That's an experience I shared, and know many others have too. That's no judgment on the women involved, far from it. It's just an indicator of how scared we are socially of this phenomenon. I recall being determined not to reveal my situation to my own NCT group, even though I was very happy to tell relative strangers. There was such a clear comparison to draw with those very particular peers, that it was too painful to mark myself out as 'other' in some way. When Joe was a bit older, and when I felt PND was now just a historical detail, I did confide in one of my NCT group, and her response was interesting:

"I'm really surprised that you had post-natal depression, I [was] always envious that you were coping so well. You always managed Joe so well, even though as you said he wasn't an easy baby. You were always doing something every day… I wish I had known because I maybe could have helped in some way."

Although she didn't know it, she did help me. The first time we met up after our babies were born, Joe was about five weeks old. It was my first proper sortie post-natally, and a very supportive friend had to chaperone me to the park because I was so anxious. When I did meet my NCT friend, her first words were, "It's really hard, isn't it?!" I was so relieved.

When Martha came to have her second child, she had a much happier experience: "I had more realistic expectations about the whole process. Possibly as a consequence, the reality was really positive. It couldn't have been more different... I felt an overwhelming rush as soon as he was born. I absolutely fell in love straight away and had goose bumps just looking at him."

For her, it was actually having such a markedly different experience second time around which confirmed her suspicion that she had had PND after her first child.

"... I didn't see my doctor about it. I thought it was just sleep deprivation. When I compare the birth of my second son, it pretty much confirms to me that I did have PND with my first. I remember going for the six week check-up with my first son and the receptionist at the GP had made an error with our booking. I didn't get seen for another four weeks. Things improved sleep-wise etc by ten weeks and so I felt better. I remember making an offhand comment to the doctor when she asked me how I felt 'in myself'. I replied that "if I had come at six weeks I would be crying by now..." I think I was hoping she would turn and say 'oh?' and she didn't. I should have asked for help, I wish I had."

Martha found it hard when other people seemed to be thriving with their new baby, but she took solace in her NCT group: "most of us were going through similar hard times." In fact, she cites making new friends as being one of the things she enjoyed about that first year. Her relationship with her mother, too, became really strong after she herself became a mum.

With her second son, she felt tired of course, and at times "overwhelmed with little things, but, by and large, it was a very happy time, if still knackering." She had new challenges, around juggling two children, and keeping the older child entertained when the baby slept to allow her some rest, but she did not feel depressed. Before he was born, she had discussed with her husband what they would do if she started to feel depressed again, and she was adamant that she would visit her doctor immediately if that transpired. But she did not have to. She reflects on what was different and points to the labour – it was much quicker and more straightforward. She credits pregnancy yoga with helping her prepare for this labour better. With two small children, she comments that yes, there were times when "I would find myself breast-feeding with one hand, getting fish fingers out of the oven for my eldest while he needed his bum wiped and the phone was ringing, and we needed to leave for nursery in ten minutes and I had had four hours sleep…" But she also remembers peaceful afternoons sitting in the park with the oldest in nursery and the baby sleeping, and she would be "feeling that life was pretty okay." She is emphatic that she feels "really, really lucky" that the second time round was such a positive experience.

5

It doesn't work like work

Jill's story

Jill is 40, and lives in Australia, where both her children (now five and one) were born.

Asked about what she thought motherhood would be like, and how the reality compared, she invokes work immediately. "At work I am incredibly competent, organised, high achieving and confident. I really expected that I would be able to deal with a baby with the same approach and skills. The reality couldn't have been more different. A small baby arrived that didn't want to be organised, didn't want to fit into a schedule, didn't want to comply with what I wanted and most of all, didn't want to sleep. I didn't really have many friends with babies and so in hindsight, I had absolutely no idea what I was in for."

Having used a private obstetrician for the birth itself, Jill didn't have a particular support network in place for afterwards. She remembers visiting midwives and lactation consultants (in Australia there is a free lactation consultation service in pharmacies), but recalls that their advice was often contradictory. Once she became aware she had PND, she did receive help from a state-run child health clinic which she still uses today. She also had support from family and close friends.

For Jill, it doesn't sound like her first birth caused her any particular trauma, she is very open about the fact that it was not as painful as she had been expecting. The labour was only around six hours, and with no time for an epidural she managed on gas and air. Her son did get stuck, and a ventouse delivery was required. Interestingly she mentions she was given an episiotomy without being told, which most people would find quite shocking, but her perspective is that it pre-empted any anxiety. She even said to her husband after the delivery "let's do that again."

She remembers feeling very happy immediately after he was placed on her chest: "it was wonderful to meet him and see what he looked like. I felt very protective of him. After the immediate birth and we were back in our hospital room, I felt quite overwhelmed and I remember thinking 'what do I do with this baby?' especially at night-time. I was amazed at how quickly I knew his smell and his sound. I could tell his cry in a ward full of babies and I remember being surprised at my physical response when he cried."

Jill was able through private health insurance to stay in hospital for three nights. This might not be right for everyone, but for her, she says, it was great, because she had 24-hour access to midwives and was able to ask them all her questions about baby care. Visiting hours were regulated, so she did not feel overwhelmed by visitors. But she was conscious of the "rigorous routine" of the ward, which she found frustrating. "Some mornings, after being awake all night with a crying baby, I'd just be climbing back into bed for some sleep and I would hear the breakfast trolley rattling down the corridor which would mean no sleep."

When she did go home, her partner had chosen not to take on work at the time, so he was around with her to help for the first four months. Nevertheless, she describes the first few weeks at home with her son as "good and bad." The couple were doing up their house, and so had not returned to the family home with their new baby, but to Jill's mother's house. Despite this meaning some living out of boxes, it sounds like she felt very supported as she had both her husband and her mum on hand, helping her look after the baby, giving her some rest, and providing comfort when she felt overwhelmed by the hormones. This was not the whole picture though. "On the other hand, it was awful. We didn't know to let him cry a little bit when we put him down for a sleep, so if he was tired, we'd put him down, as soon as he cried, we'd pick him up, so we thought he would never sleep and we were just making him more and more tired and ourselves more stressed. The nights were particularly awful for me. I'd get up to breast-feed during the night, it was winter, it was freezing (no central heating in Australia) and I was alone. For some strange reason, I don't know why I did it now, but I would attempt to rock the baby back to sleep after each feed and he would take forever to fall asleep and then not sleep for longer than one sleep cycle. I'd then get him up, feed him again, rock him to sleep again… it was endless. I remember standing at the window rocking this baby and watching dawn approach, the sun start to rise and then the bright light of morning would be there and I wouldn't have slept a wink for most of the night. It was the worst time of my life (so far). I developed an absolute dread of being on my own after that, which took me a long time to overcome."

Jill's description of what it felt like developing PND is very vivid:

"…like drowning but still being alive at the same time… A dreadful feeling of sinking down under a sea of black water, not being able to breathe, not being able to swim back up to the top, screaming to be heard but nobody could hear you under the black water, of being surrounded by people but nobody could see or hear you. I used to go to bed at night, pull all the heavy blankets over my head and hope and pray that I died during the night and was so disappointed when I woke up... My PND got so bad I considered self-harming. I wanted to dig my fingernails into my scalp and then claw all the way down the sides of my face. As a compromise I started tearing at the skin on my wrists with my fingernails. This is actually quite painful so I gave that up. I would wish I was dead and think about suicide in general, but no specific thoughts about actually killing myself. I felt like I was such a mess that I was sure my baby would be better off without me." She says her PND peaked when her son was ten to 12 weeks old.

A visit to her GP involved a long consultation and several questionnaires, after which they concluded together that she had PND. A plan was drawn up, which included six appointments with a psychologist. Jill didn't like the first one she saw, but found the second one to be excellent, and very helpful. She was taught to recognise and accept her feelings about motherhood. She was also shown how to reappraise her preconceptions about the perfect mother. The relationship has continued intermittently, and she still sees her occasionally when things become overwhelming. She was prescribed anti-depressants but resisted taking them due to breast-feeding. I wondered if she was told they were unsafe – because I know that there are certainly anti-depressants which are safe during breast-feeding. But she also said that she was worried she would feel too good if she took them

– that she would not want to stop, and mentioned this has happened to some of her friends.

Jill also credits her local (free) child health clinic with her recovery. She developed a very strong relationship with three nurses working there, who she still sees with her second son. They helped her on sleep issues, which she feels were big factors in her depression. "Because of my depression and potential for self-harm, the nurses were able to fast-track my acceptance into a government-provided residential sleep clinic for mums and bubs. This was one of the best things I have ever done. My son was eight months old when we went to the sleep clinic and I learned so much. I wish it was compulsory for all new mums to go to such a centre and I wish I hadn't waited so long to ask for help."

Looking back, it is apparent to her that there were a lot of circumstances at play when she developed PND. Within a month she had moved house, left a job she loved, started renovating the family home and had her first baby. She feels now that this was clearly too much change, too soon. But it is not something she could have been averted from: she was confident she could handle it all.

"I found my baby's sleep the most challenging aspect of being a new mum. He didn't sleep, I didn't know why, I couldn't get him to sleep, etc. I also found the cluster-feeding in the early part of the evening very demanding too, just when I was my most tired, my most hungry and most emotional my baby was being the most demanding."

Having recently moved, Jill was far away from her close friends. She did quickly meet "mum friends" through a local group, which helped. But her main relationship: with her husband, was hugely affected. They had been together over a decade before their first child arrived, and suddenly everything was different. She feels that her husband probably could not understand why she was unable to cope, and this drove a wedge between the couple.

Throughout the period of having PND, she was able to feel moments of happiness, and was grateful for having her son, because it had taken the couple longer than they had expected to have a baby. Once the PND had begun to wane, she took pleasure in watching her child grow and develop, and she enjoyed making new friends. But some time after she recovered from PND, she found herself developing depression again.

"I missed working, missed having a purpose in life other than being a mum, missed being in control of things, and missed feeling the highs that a 'high achiever' (as I was at work) likes to feel. Some more visits to my psychologist helped with this. I also went back to work three days a week."

Three and a half years after having her first son, she had another son. The couple suffered three miscarriages in the interim. When Jill got pregnant again she was very aware of the possibility of having PND again. "I knew what PND 'felt' like and so I was very aware of recognising the feelings and symptoms of PND and dealing with them very quickly. I understood the importance of maintaining my support network and relying on them as often as necessary and being very truthful about how I was feeling. I also knew I couldn't rely on my husband to help me through another round of PND and so I bypassed him and went to other support network members. I definitely feel like I did have a mild case of PND with my second child, however I was much better equipped to recognise it and deal with it. I knew so much more about baby sleep issues so I think this was a big contributor to my depression not being so big or lasting so long."

Like many mothers after having a second child, Jill found the initial juggling act quite challenging. She says that it was impossible to get both children to nap at the same time, so she struggled to get rest herself. Then when her younger son was three months old he became very ill, which really affected his sleep over the following four months. She found his illness traumatic, and the sleep deprivation made coping even harder. But the age gap was manageable, and in many ways her older son was able to understand the demands the new baby was placing on his mother, and to entertain himself for instance when she was breast-feeding.

Today, she feels like she has left PND behind and moved on. But what does linger is the resentment caused by what she felt was a lack of understanding from her husband when she was going through depression. She can't escape the feeling that he let her down, though she questions if this is a fair reaction from her. However, it is also a brave and honest one. Her advice is not to rely on just one person to get through PND. She thinks it is sensible to identify a group of friends you know you can rely on, as well as contacting relevant health professionals. "Take anti-depressants if you really need to," she adds.

Jill now encourages friends to be honest about how they feel in the same situation; "there are no right or wrong feelings". She thinks mothers need to ask for help straightaway, and says "motherhood is not a wonderful experience all day every day for some of us, and that's okay." She believes the more honest we are, the more we can chip away at the stigma which surrounds PND, which should lead to women asking for help more readily. "This can only be a good thing for our mums first and foremost, and for their bubs."

6

My PND with #1 continued…

I don't know why I ended up with post-natal depression with my first child. Second time around I was prepared for it, because I know it was more likely, given I'd had it once. But with my first son, there were certainly a series of external circumstances which must have been factors.

I had planned a home birth, having had a very straightforward pregnancy. A friend had had one, and despite significant scepticism from some quarters, I was convinced that it was a good plan. I made this decision – with Ben's agreement, and a supportive midwife – in North London, but at about 20 weeks we moved to South London, to an area which, if anything, is even more pro-home births judging by the number of people who seem to have had them. But suddenly at about 34 weeks I was diagnosed with pre-eclampsia. I suppose in hindsight, my blood pressure had been steadily climbing, but having moved half way through the pregnancy there was perhaps some inconsistency in my notes. I remember feeling very stressed at work – I put myself under a lot of pressure, unnecessarily so, because my employers were always very understanding. After I left my first NCT class, I flicked through the free magazine we had been given, on the train into work. I noticed an article stating that one of the warning signs of pre-eclampsia was headaches with flashing lights. I'd had this the previous week, but somehow among all my reading, I had missed what it could be a sign of. I immediately got checked out, but initially was not diagnosed with pre-eclampsia – this came later, after a particularly unglamorous 24 hour urine test during a stay in hospital.

Like many people, I have a horror of hospital stays, for me probably partly because I had a particularly traumatic one following a botched termination in my 20s. As luck would have it, I was now in the same hospital, feeling confused, not very well, and anxious about my planned birth, which I was now told (albeit gently) would need to take place in the (same) hospital, rather than at home. A scan revealed that Joe had stopped growing in the womb. Although he seemed 'happy', the conclusion was a likely induction and delivery at 37 weeks, and I was signed off work.

A couple of days essentially in limbo followed, then suddenly and spontaneously my waters broke of their own accord at 36 weeks and five days, and he was born a day later – so only technically one day premature – at a small but healthy 5 lbs 4 oz. It's only now, having talked to several mental health professionals while writing this book, that I think it's possible I had post traumatic stress disorder following Joe's birth. It started as a straightforward labour, I managed contractions "well" according to the midwife, and in fact she had been surprised, on an examination at home, to find I was already about five centimetres dilated, so I was transferred to hospital. I say transferred – this involved an excruciating ten minute car journey with Ben at the wheel, and me thinking, "I

NEVER want to do this again" – which of course I would, two years and seven months later, this time in an ambulance. For some reason though, once in hospital, and once things got to the stage where I was supposed to be pushing – perhaps because of his small size – Joe appeared to get stuck. In an email I sent to someone I was mentoring 18 months later, when we were swapping stories, I said, "it all ended up being traumatic, with my blood pressure shooting up and his heart rate dipping. So I was rushed to theatre, where they prepped me for C-section but in the end he came very easily with forceps. I found this all quite shocking I think - it suddenly took a very different course." I remember still having flashing lights and headaches in the minutes after I gave birth, but nobody really seemed to register this.

The week that followed, as I have already said, was probably the worst of my life. I've had a pretty good life, but that's still saying something. Joe's weight, coupled with low blood sugar, meant we were on a strict feeding regime from the start – yet breast-feeding was a nightmare, and just didn't happen. There seemed to be no contingency for this (like, say formula?!). We were cup-feeding him donor breast milk instead. I've since found many other women who experienced the dreaded cups. They spill the milk everywhere (particularly maddening if it's milk you've wearily expressed yourself, you really do cry over spilt milk then). Even though I'd been told by everyone that "birth would cure" the pre-eclampsia, I became quite ill in the days following the birth. We subsequently found out that the few days after birth can be very high risk for eclampsia. By the time the staff, who were rushed off their feet, realised that it was more than just usual new mum tiredness and anxiety, it took days to find the right treatment for my blood pressure. At one stage

I became breathless, only to find that I had wrongly been prescribed a drug which should not be taken by asthmatics, which I am. Like so many women I know and have talked to, my story involves watching the clock – wishing the night would pass, trying and failing to comfort a screaming baby (who, in retrospect, I realise was probably just hungry), waiting till the earliest point my husband was allowed back in, like visiting hours in prison. Nobody was available to help me at night, understandably in a busy London hospital, but regrettably, because I did not sleep all week. The donor milk would run out, and of course nobody wanted to suggest formula. We, in our sleep-deprived, befuddled states, just didn't think of it.

When we finally got home, we were kind of shell-shocked. Everyone else's stories of those early days were so far from my experience. I'd hoped to slot into the life my friends who had had babies had experienced, living with their newborns, but it just didn't happen. I felt crippled with anxiety about leaving the house, I sobbed all the time - and knew it was more than baby blues, and the fact that the feeding didn't happen felt very awkward because it seemed to me that the community I was living in was breast feeding central. I had never considered it wouldn't work for me. I fully support a mother's right and even her need to breast-feed, and feel fortunate to live in an area with so much support on offer to fulfill that – but sometimes it can be overwhelming knowing which way to turn. I could fill a separate book on the breastfeeding issue, and it is an area fraught with tension, because the main players have a huge emotional interest in it. For me, perhaps we could have succeeded, but at two weeks in and on my knees with exhaustion, depression and a very hungry baby, I threw the towel in. My midwives were surprisingly supportive of that decision; I think they could see how desperate I was. In fact our main midwife described us on our first night home as "a couple on the edge". We then had various health issues with my son - none of them major but enough to require various trips to A&E and then Great Ormond Street, all very stressful at just a few weeks of age.

I constantly asked my husband why we'd ruined our happy life by having a baby. To make matters more fraught, he was never an easy baby, or so it seemed to me - he was a screamer, it felt to me as though he was the only baby who wasn't all sleepy cuddles and milky grins. I know to some on the natural motherhood end, that talk of 'easy babies' is anathema. But it's important to remember that all of this was happening through the prism of depression. All I could see was what I thought was going wrong.

I knew all along it wasn't just baby blues. I remember crying and crying in hospital, and knowing this was not going to go away. At about four weeks in, I saw the doctor and did the Edinburgh Scale questionnaire to diagnose post-natal depression - the results were pretty unequivocal; I think I scored about 21 out of 25, 25 being extremely depressed. She prescribed me anti-depressants and a course of counselling.

And the sense of something lifting was palpable. Of course it didn't go away overnight, and, for instance, the eight sessions of counselling were arguably as helpful as the drugs. My husband's advice was always "do what you need to do, when you need to – and when you're able to." He said this because he knew I was constantly comparing myself to the other new mums I could see gadding about. My perception was that I was inadequate. So I created a life which involved manageable things: slowly building a network of friends over time, rather than rushing around in a sort of Freshers' week-style frenzy, trying to get to know every new mum in the area.

I was quite circumspect, probably partly because I had PND and didn't feel very comfortable blurting that out to strangers. For me a session which worked was the local library rhyme time. Here I could be as social as I wanted to, but there was no obligation or even real opportunity to chat to anyone else. Really it was about learning songs to sing to my baby. As is probably clear by now, I had real problems bonding with my first son. I could see objectively that he was very sweet, and I knew rationally I ought to be happy, but I felt oddly detached, and sometimes the strongest sensation I had was one of *inconvenience*. The seemingly small step of learning some songs to sing to him, and using them to calm him when I needed to, really helped me to build a connection with him. Another deceptively simple, and apparently basic step was just getting outside. For whatever reason, fresh air helped. It was very difficult to break out of the cycle of staying in the house – hiding – for hours on end, watching another episode of Gilmour Girls; the afternoons in the dark room with the remote were stultifying. And probably weren't helping with the missing bond either. What I credit the anti-depressants with is giving me the ability to actually get out of the house, and overcome some of that irrational anxiety – what if he cries, what if I run out of formula, what if he needs changing and there isn't a baby-change – enabling me to get out of the house, which in turn always, always lifted my spirits.

We are fortunate to live in an area of London with a great choice of parks and green spaces. Though I don't now live so near the park I used to visit when Joe was a baby, every time I go back there I am transported right back to my first tentative walk there when he was five weeks old. I still feel emotional at times, remembering how just walking across that open space was incredibly uplifting and liberating.

7

PND, the sequel

Given everything I have recorded about my first bout of PND, you'd think we might have learned something. But we went into having a second child telling ourselves, "we are so much wiser now! We'll be so much more relaxed! And some stuff that worked, we'll do that again. And the stuff that didn't work, we'll do it differently. And, voila!"

Just like with baby number one, everyone spouts complete falsehoods about second babies. Oh, it's so much easier. That would be true if you subtracted the first child from the equation. And if the second child was *exactly like* the first child so that all your "lessons learned" could be applied. Oh, the second one just fits in, and sleeps through anything. No, no he didn't. Number two had severe reflux. After a two week honeymoon period, this kicked in and suddenly all our proclamations that number one had been a difficult baby seemed wildly inaccurate. Number two was a banshee. I had my two weeks of just enjoying him and even managing to breast-feed, in combination with formula. But almost overnight, as reflux took serious hold, he changed. One lesson learned that did help was that we got specialist help straight away. We did not mess around. And that helped enormously. Likewise, as soon as I recognised I was falling into the PND pit all over again, I went to my GP and said, "I have post-natal depression, I'd like Sertraline again and I'd like to be referred for CBT". So that was one small voila, I will give you that. In fact, looking back, I realise that even before he started showing reflux signs, I was showing my own signs of retreading the PND path. I remember feeling absurdly anxious about leaving the house with both children. And the night before my husband went back to work after paternity leave, I had a panic attack. I spent that first day inside with both kids, wondering if I would ever leave the house again. Nonetheless, PND second time around was at least a known quantity. When Ted was 11 days old I sent an email to a friend, saying:

"I think though that even when things seem tough - and have def had some of those dark cloud moments which you probably remember - at least I kind of know what I'm dealing with, so am fully prepared to go for the drugs/counselling if I feel I need it, though so far think am fine as long as I get some sleep/food!"

Then a week later, I said:

"Mum is coming back down tonight as have been struggling. Some bits going well, other moments absolutely awful, and hate having all the same feelings I had with Joe (that I've made a mistake, was mad to think could handle two etc). Ben is helping loads which means I'm getting some sleep which does make a difference. Hopefully the drugs will kick in soon…

… Sometimes everything seems v manageable and do-able, other times the complete opposite and [I] feel completely hopeless."

By the time Ted was a month old, I was sending regular despairing bulletins to my husband: "… sigh. Joe has had about five hours TV. Ted sleeping during feeds still. Not sure how to turn either of these things around."

Somewhere in between, I'd made that visit to the GP. And a few days later, I was emailing that my mum (who had been staying with us) was worried about returning home to Scotland, because of how things were going. Oddly at this distance of three years on, I can barely remember, but it seems Ted's problems with feeding were all-consuming, leading to a bizarre 'split feed' arrangement which obviously wasn't conducive to managing the needs of a highly active two and a half year old. All those reassurances that things would be easier, that he would just fit in; not for us, the healing second time round.

But were we not the most to blame? Had we fallen into the same trap all over again? Thinking we could impose our will, our needs, our structure onto a newborn? Is the biggest lesson of all that we are personally, and perhaps more widely, generationally, selfish? Out of touch with what parenting is really all about?

A few days later I emailed a friend:

"Mum here till Thursday as I've still not been getting better on the drugs, and sleep got a whole lot worse in the last few nights. Which of course makes things seem more bleak. Ted has bad reflux and Gaviscon not helping - he wakes himself up being sick after 45 mins -1 hour of sleep and screaming, so nights have not been fun at all. Going to the doc again today to demand specialist referral which is what we should have done with Joe - all that screaming I now think was prob his reflux - not going to let that happen again. Have been on the drugs [Sertraline] three weeks - they give it six before they will up dose or change medication. Again though I would like a specialist to see me as [my] GPs know nothing about depression it seems. Just tell me to make some mummy friends and go to baby groups - ARGH! I have friends! It's just that when things are bad I feel disconnected from everyone. Even Ben.

Joe is also playing up a lot, because he knows he can I guess. Quite nervous about mum going away again but can't expect her to stay forever. But she's already extended her stay a few times as she's been quite worried."

And a week later I followed this up:

"... has been good having mum as particularly with the lack of sleep, it is hard to function when feeling so crap, and hard enough in the early weeks anyway. It is just SO tedious being depressed, there's not even any point talking about it with anyone as it just is what it is, and you just have to hope it goes soon. I do hate how crippling it is, makes me feel v incapable and I look at how well others manage with one, two or even three kids and feel a bit inadequate. Did have a good debrief with the midwife from the birth yesterday, who basically said I was unlucky with the birth (in terms of the things that went wrong) and she felt I had a particularly painful labour, so that made me feel a bit better about going to pieces during it!"

I also documented my suspicion that I'd been fobbed off in one of my early attempts to address Ted's reflux, because the GP had noticed the PND diagnosis in my notes.

For the record, as well as sending all these slightly desperate missives, I received many supportive emails, among them this reply to the email above, from a dear friend. I remember this really did help. And I hope the sentiment might help others too:

"... And when you're feeling like other people cope better, remember that a lot of people are very selective about what they reveal and it's also not a level playing field. Some people have both mums around, or husbands at home, or ridiculously easy babies... or no PND. You are at one of the toughest ends of it. Your mum isn't on your doorstep long term, Ben's in an office, Ted cries all night and Joe is a usual hyperactive toddler who can't possibly understand what's going on. And you're suffering proper proper depression. Be generous to yourself and try not to compare things to other people. I know you know this, but I know that I appreciate verification so I hope you do."

The point about comparisons is an ongoing thread in my experience as a parent. The motto of a friend's father -- originally coined by Evelyn Waugh in A Handful of Dust - was introduced to me in this context some time ago, and I find it very helpful: "comparisons are odious." Isn't that great? It is so easy to look around constantly, noticing seemingly wonderful parents, particularly mums, spinning dozens of plates and looking fabulous while they do it. I know that comparisons are odious. But I do need to remind myself. Because even now, six years after my first experience of motherhood, I catch myself benchmarking. I receive a thank you card from a friend for a new baby present - just days after I sent the present. My first thought (after noting of course that her new baby was beautiful) is "I didn't get round to thank you cards till Joe was at least three months old!" This is not a particularly attractive trait. And it's also not at all constructive. But it is compulsive. One of the lessons I learned in CBT was that the well-trodden path the mind takes when we are thinking negatively – is the "easy" path. And what we need to do is work to take the less obvious path. So the aim is not to think, "I'm sure I wasn't coping as well as her…", but to try to think, "good for her!" and remember those many times when people would comment on something that you were handling well, the way it perhaps seemed to the outside world, the pub lunch when four week old Joe slept for three hours and everyone commented on how well we were getting on. The reality was for those three hours I probably had forgotten he existed, and was in a bubble pretending my life had not changed.

Annie's story

PND is nothing if not an unpredictable beast. Embittered though I may feel that I fell into the "more likely to recur" bracket of PND with baby number two, I know many women have several children and only experience it once, which is something worth remembering given how many women who have it once become very afraid of developing it again.

Annie has three children, and had PND after her second child was born, though it was not diagnosed. She estimates that it peaked when her second child was six to eight months old. Before having children, Annie had a successful career in television, working long hours. She says that she had few expectations of motherhood "which the first time around was a huge help I discovered, as there was no clash of vision versus reality. The only thing I expected when I was pregnant with my first child was to enjoy their company and relish the chance to be off work and both panned out."

I include Annie's story here for many reasons, one of them being that she had positive birth experiences with each of her three children. She is open about the fact that she was fortunate to be able to afford some private healthcare which she believes offered her a level of care which, really, women should expect on the NHS. With her first child, she describes the birth as:

"Perfect. It was exactly as I had wished it to be and then some. I had an elective C-section and it all went really smoothly. I was also lucky to recover really quickly. My main memory of his birth is feeling utterly elated."

I think it's important to share this part of her story, because there is often such a premium put on natural birth (even if just by the mothers themselves) – but she exemplifies the fact that a C-section can be equally positive. Perhaps as a result of this experience, Annie bonded straightaway with her first child, a little boy. She had a five day stay in hospital after the birth, but says, "It was a private hospital, so this was enjoyable. I wish to god the NHS could provide the maternity care that the private sector offers as women would be so better served. The key differences that made those first days go smoothly and that you can't expect on the NHS were: continuity of care - the same midwife from birth to going home; flexible visiting hours and the ability to have your partner sleep in your room; food that is actually edible; excellent breastfeeding support; your own room; a nursery facility that allows you to sleep when your baby is sleeping and midwives to help you learn how to bathe, feed and dress your baby. Also daily visits from a paediatrician to answer all the questions any anxious first time parent has."

Annie also describes a solid support network: her mother, mother-in-law and sister were all very hands on during the first two months of her son's life. Her husband during that time worked part-time, and from home, so was actively co-parenting. Overall, she says that period was "blissful", though there were low moments. She says that she enjoyed being at home, and having time to herself, having spent a decade in a frantic work environment. "At first I couldn't understand all those mums who said they didn't have time to shower or read or cook. I felt I'd never had MORE time to myself." This was because her son was asleep throughout much of the day, so she was able to enjoy being at home. There was a pay-off though: "he slept very badly at night, but we were so naïve that we thought it was normal and weren't overly stressed by it… We were a happy unit and I enjoyed the company of my son and myself so I failed to create a network of local mums which was something that led later to loneliness and a feeling of isolation when PND hit after baby two." She describes herself as being "utterly in love" with her first child from the start.

With her second, Annie had a different experience post-natally. By her own admission, she had expected everything would go the same way it had first time around. But, it didn't, which:

"caused… huge amounts of anxiety, frustration, and, at times, anger. On the plus side, it gave me the tools to truly empathise with friends who had found motherhood difficult and alienating. And for me, that is a real silver lining to the cloud of post-natal depression that I suffered after having my second child."

For various reasons, the support which had been so comprehensive first time around couldn't be there on the same level after her second child, yet ironically she felt much more in need of it. The reality of juggling a newborn and a two year old was very challenging. This was a contrast to first time around.

"After my second child was born I expected to be thrown back into the same euphoric state that I had felt after having my first child. Almost immediately things felt different. I was riddled with irrational concerns. My new baby had an 'outie' belly button and I was convinced that this was a really, really bad thing. That her life would be marred. That it must have been my fault. Did I have too much wine one night? Was it eating the wrong cheese? It was completely and utterly irrational and a small part of me knew it but I was overwhelmed by feeling this was somehow a failure."

She also felt angry a lot of the time:

"I took to shouting at my husband all the time. Nothing he could do was enough and everything he did do, he did wrong. Or so I thought. Our first child was right in the 'terrible twos' and the multiple tantrums on a daily basis made me boil with rage. I couldn't connect with him in the way I wanted to. It was SO much effort to be kind and respectful."

But what she says was the "really awful part" was the intrusive thoughts she experienced.

"All I thought about was dying. I felt that I was in a battle to survive with my new baby. That it was her or me. Initially I had very violent thoughts towards her. I thought how easy it would be to kill her. But that phase was brief. I decided early on that it made more sense if I just went. And by 'went' I mean die. So I focused on preparing the family to cope without me. And when it looked like they couldn't I was furious. If my husband put their clothes on the wrong way or gave them the wrong food or let them play with toys that weren't safe or left the washing machine door open I would go crazy. And it all became so normal to me that I would take to accusing him of making it impossible for me to die. I didn't realise the madness of what I was saying. It was utterly logical to me. I wanted to go but I wanted to go knowing they would be looked after."

To compound matters, Annie's new baby would not take a bottle, so she felt "chained to her... there was no respite. No one else could get up in the night or take her for a few hours. And it meant that dying was not an option as I needed her to be able to be fed. We had midwives, health visitors and eventually very expensive specialist nannies to assist and no one could get her to take a bottle. In the end, I suppose this saved me."

Annie says she felt very isolated: "I was hit by the loneliness", with no nearby friends or family when her second child was small. She also felt that she would never recover her former career fully, so she needed to think about who she was beyond being a mother. Without a formal diagnosis, she had no support beyond her husband, who was the only person she confided in – she swore him to secrecy.

Part of the problem with her second experience of motherhood was the juggling. "The adjustment from one to two children felt more like going from one to five. I couldn't cope at all. I had a two year old who was, to all intents and purposes, a baby still and this new baby who demanded even more attention. Both slept terribly and I was shattered."

I was stunned by her description of what had happened to her, and very interested to know how she coped. I met up with her to talk about it more, and asked her about "masking" – which she had been exceptional at. Her husband alone knew the extent of it, not least because he was often the focus. I wondered how had she managed to dig herself out of that hole, with no outside help? I don't think she would ever suggest another person should do the same: when I ask her what advice she would have for someone in the same situation, she says without hesitation, "Don't keep it in. Try, try, try to share what you are going through." I wondered why she didn't seek help, since she knew on some level that her behaviour was irrational. She said that it was the same fear everyone has: what if they take the children away?

I pressed Annie on what had helped her to get out of the depression. She says, "I don't think there was a lightbulb moment when I realised that the cloud had passed. It was gradual and definitely linked to getting the baby in a better sleep pattern."

When her daughter was around eight months old, and things had reached a really low point, she and her husband discussed what their strategy should be to improve things. They knew they had to do something. They conceded defeat on the bottle, but considered what else they could do to help things. Attempts to go out for an evening always led to a call from her husband or babysitter with a screaming baby in the background, begging her to return so she could be fed. "I felt so imprisoned," she says. The couple realised that if they could improve their baby's sleep, Annie stood a chance of having some time to herself in the evening. So they focused on trying to improve her sleeping routine. Things started to improve once she was regularly going down for the evening at 7pm. "She wouldn't sleep all night, but enough that we could go out for dinner and a movie or see friends." The couple also felt they needed some respite at this stage, for the sake of their marriage. When their daughter was just over a year old, they had the chance to attend a friend's wedding overseas. "We jumped at it. In the run up, we'd got her to successfully take just enough milk from a cup and sleep right through the night. Our mothers agreed to split the childcare and then a miracle happened - a few days before we went she started to drink from a bottle. As a result we went off with a huge weight lifted from our shoulders. We had a baby who, at last, slept through the night and could be soothed and settled by someone other than me."

The couple were away for a week, and she describes it as "the final step to recovery... [spending time] with just my husband and remembering the reasons that we'd had babies and pledged to spend our life together. I think we had forgotten how to be kind and considerate and loving to each other. Every day had just felt like a battle to survive and we had sharpened our elbows to each other. Vicious arguments about who was more sleep deprived, who was more miserable, who was more in need of a night out. But here we could both be out late, both sleep late... and eat in restaurants that don't have high chairs or kids menu! It levelled us and brought us back together. And when we got home we felt hopeful and happy at last."

I asked her, as I've asked everyone, whether she considered medication.

"I considered taking anti-depressants a lot and it was a bad decision not to. I was obsessed with being branded a mad lady and on the radar of social services and it defied all logic as I have friends who have been successfully treated for depression with medication and should they have ever asked for my opinion before taking them I would have absolutely encouraged it and told them that their concerns were silly. I was keen on therapy and explored this as a route."

She doesn't think any of the healthcare professionals she dealt with regularly – GP, midwives, health visitors – had any idea of what she was going through, saying she was very good at putting a happy face on "when it mattered. Not quite Oscar-worthy but up there!"

Initially, Annie's experience after her second child put her and her husband off having further children. Her husband in particular felt the risks were too high. "We both feel I came very close to doing something disastrous and I was sad as I had hoped for three children but accepted that this made sense." Then she got pregnant by accident. At first, the couple were shocked and devastated by this news. "My husband thought it would be the end of us. It took a long time to accept but we went ahead and planned for it." The couple made sure that they would have additional support after the birth of baby number three. A post-natal doula came in every morning for the first month to help. "And it helped. It really, really made the difference... I think it made the first few weeks so much easier to have all that support." In addition, the new baby has been very easy – sleeping well, crying little, feeding easily. She too doesn't take a bottle, but because this time around Annie is not depressed and feels supported, she has found she can handle it.

Her additional advice to others: "People want to help. They really do and if you let them in it will make all the difference."

"I want people to know that while one case of PND means you have a greater likelihood of having it again, it doesn't mean you WILL have it again. I didn't and I am so glad now that I had another child after PND. Also, don't just know that help is there. Go find it. Take a deep breath and tell a trusted friend or family member. Once you have made that first move the rest will be much easier. It does leave you. It might not feel it - in fact it probably won't feel it - but it will."

8

… but for me it was recurring

PND second time around for me was far less clear-cut
than the first time, when it defined everything about that
first year. Second time, particularly in hindsight, it is hard to
tell where the PND ended and general ennui of family life,
of juggling the demands of two differently aged children,
began. Certainly when I think and talk about PND it is the
experience with Joe which I return to again and again. Second
time around there was a feeling of, "I know this one…"
and once I'd sought diagnosis, treatment and counselling,
I felt I had dispatched it – which of course was not exactly
true. The key difference in how I reacted the second time
was that I sought CBT. I had heard through many people,
particularly one of the case studies described in this book,
a young woman I informally 'mentored' through PND, that
CBT was incredibly effective at helping to manage some of
the symptoms of PND. I was fortunate to be fast-tracked for
specialist help, in line with NICE guidelines.

After an assessment with a psychologist, I was referred
for CBT. I was initially told I'd receive up to six appointments
with my therapist, on a strictly weekly basis (i.e. missing a

week was strongly discouraged). In the end I was seen for around nine months. I have since discussed CBT with other women who suffered from PND, and not all found it helpful. I imagine it is much to do with the individual you are seen by. I was fortunate to have someone I liked, and who 'got' me, based at the nearby Maudsley hospital – an incredible resource I feel very fortunate to have on my doorstep. We made a breakthrough when we discussed perfectionism – not, as I'd previously thought, mutually exclusive from people who are not especially house-proud – and moved on to assertiveness. Although initially unsure – was this really going to help with PND – I went with it, and found that issues which pre-dated my children being born were affecting the way I handled being a mother. So, for example, lack of assertiveness meant I struggled to cope with strong characters telling me what to do with my baby. It meant I was scared of people in authority and how to push for what I felt I needed for myself and my family. It meant I said 'yes' to too many things, when I should have said 'no', and so banked lots of bonus stress for myself.

The perfectionism thing was interesting. How could I be a perfectionist when I couldn't care less how messy my house was? When I was happy to leave the house with a top my infant son had just casually sprinkled with pee? What I learned was that perfectionism takes many forms. For me, I *had* to know that my son's schedule would be adhered to. I *had* to know that something would go well before I entertained the idea of doing it. So – first time around at least - going to a baby group was terrifying: what if he cried? What if he needed a feed or new nappy and I couldn't handle it? Meeting up with mummy friends was bound up with similar fears. What if I should host, what then? What if I didn't have the right food? If I get brownies from the bakery, what if someone has a nut allergy? When they come and their babies are all more perfect and easy than mine, what if they judge me? What if it makes me feel worse? The option of staying at home, of seeing nobody was always easier. Second time around I became obsessed with the stress of hosting playdates, or even attending them, because my older son would throw tantrums and I was convinced everyone thought of him as *that* child, but I was so tired and stressed with the baby I didn't feel equipped to handle it. I remember having long conversations with my therapist about what food would be acceptable to serve for tea if I was hosting a playdate. Typing this feels faintly ridiculous (now with a child nearing his second year of school, I have significantly lowered my standards when it comes to playdates). But it's an example of how things played on my mind.

Choosing to just stay in wasn't an option with an energetic two year old, but it had been when he was my only baby. After one frenzied reading of Secrets of the Baby Whisperer, when my first son was tiny, I listed my time as recommended in the book. This follows the E-A-S-Y routine: Eat, Activity, Sleep, YOU, i.e., when the baby sleeps, take some time for yourself. I diligently kept a diary for a day or two chronicling my adherence to this regime. Under "You"' I wrote "Prison Break". This referred to the fact that I was working my way through a box set of the series. My mum, reading the note, misunderstood and said very seriously, "it does feel like breaking out of prison when you get out doesn't it?" It still makes me laugh, this comic misunderstanding, the well-meaning solicitude of my mum, the fact that although she got it wrong, she also sort of got it right. It was like prison. But the really sad thing is I thought I was having 'me time', by staying in and watching a programme I liked. But I was hiding. I thought I was escaping. I was keeping myself in prison without even realising.

When I had my second son, a friend who was incredibly supportive to me during my first experience of post-natal depression visited and, seeing how challenging I was finding things with the two children, commented that she really hoped I wouldn't hole up at home again, the way I had first time around. She quite rightly identified that being outside, in fresh air, getting sunlight and a bit of exercise – as well as the enormous confidence boost of *managing* it – would be good for me. But sometimes just making the step, the step you know will help, is too hard. I've already documented how my doctor told me anti-depressants would help me to take that step – and, thankfully, she was right. I don't suggest medication is the panacea. Nor is it right for everybody. I just, rather selfishly I suppose, feel so thankful that it worked for me.

So now, after two babies and two episodes of post-natal depression, I knew a bit more about perfectionism and the part it played. What could I do about it? My therapist introduced me to a concept I have quoted ad nauseam ever since, and shared with many friends – to the extent that it's now a running joke between myself, my husband, my mum and several close friends. "Dare to be average," she encouraged me. She referred me to a chapter of a book by psychiatrist David Burns. He writes in his book, *Feeling Good: The New Mood Therapy*, that he took up jogging in the 1970s. As I knew he had a beard, since I read this bit I have forever pictured him as one of the 118 118 joggers, which is slightly unfortunate. But although the jogging example is a little of its time, his point is brilliant. He writes that he took up jogging, and after becoming frustrated with his progress, he inverted the usual approach an athlete would take. Instead of trying to beat his time each day, he aimed to do *worse*, to fall short of his personal best. This way, if he exceeded his previous best, that was of course a massive bonus. But if he fell short of it, that was what he had aimed for, nothing to lament. He puts this concept into an academic context, saying that if one aims only to be the best, to get the top grade, we will at very best just feel ambivalent – best case scenario, we got what we were aiming for. We can never exceed those hopes. When we consider this, it's actually quite depressing. If we stop trying to be flawless, anything we do is going to feel like an achievement.

I wish I'd discovered this idea when I had my first child. It's become my motto. It's simple and incredibly liberating. I know I err towards not trying things if I suspect I won't be able to master them, or do them well. I also blame myself if something isn't *just right*, and can worry about an event for days just anticipating how and where I may fall short of 'full marks'. If you add this tendency to a work context, it's a hindrance. If you add it to the context of someone who has just become a mother, it is debilitating.

9

PND is not the only player... PTSD, anxiety and other players

Sarah's story

When Joe was about nine months old, and my depression had all but completely receded, I was put in touch with a friend of a friend who had recently been diagnosed with PND. The mutual friend was looking for ways to support her. I offered to email or meet with the friend, since that was something I had found helpful when I was in the midst of the dark days myself. The friend put me in touch with Sarah, whose son was then four months old. We started emailing, and occasionally meeting up. Reviewing our early emails has been a startling reminder of how I felt back then, and is as good as any description of what the early days of PND were like, written only a few months later when everything was still so fresh in my mind. I wrote to her:

"... you've got a baby about six weeks and have been diagnosed with PND - I was too at about the same time - so thought it might be useful to 'talk' on email..." I explained the circumstances of Joe's birth, and then continued: "Right from about day two - having had no sleep on the first night as Joe wouldn't sleep unless he was held - I started crying a lot. This went on and on for weeks, so that what I'd initially dismissed as 'baby blues' and exhaustion, became more and more obviously something a bit more serious. The kinds of things going through my head were 'I don't want to do this... what have I done... I just want it to be me and my husband again'. I don't mean to say I wished Joe away - it was almost that I just wished someone else could look after him. I felt as though an earthquake had happened in my life and none of it made sense any more, even though I could function in some ways - send emails, deal with the baby (even when it felt like I was doing a crap job). I found though that my midwives and people in general were reluctant to talk about PND that early on. In the end I went to see my GP with my husband in tow for back up and basically had hysterics in the doctor's surgery. I was referred to a different GP who specialises in post-natal stuff, and she did the 'Edinburgh Scale' quiz with me - have you done this? She referred me to a counsellor attached to the surgery who I saw in the end for eight sessions and which I'd highly recommend. At the time I was like, I can talk to my husband, my friends, why do I need a counsellor? I wanted someone to tell me what to do, not someone to listen to me. But actually it was brilliant - it helped me to sort through so much stuff. She (my GP) also prescribed anti-depressants which I held off taking for a week and then after one spectacular meltdown where I called my husband sobbing that I couldn't physically go on, I started taking them! I can honestly say I think that's what turned everything around. It was a slow process but I remember noticing that whole days would go by when I didn't cry... then weeks... my GP summed up what the drugs do very well; she said they won't make it all go away, but they will give you the 'ooomph' to get out and do things, and the getting out etc will be what lifts your mood. They certainly seemed to help me cope - that was the big stumbling block for me before hand, I just constantly felt overwhelmed. I also had this catch 22 situation where I would go mad being in (it was winter and plus I'd been told not to take Joe out till he was a bit stronger) all day but I felt crippled with fear about going anywhere. I think part of this was having had the first week in hospital, and part was because I couldn't breast-feed so I got obsessed about being out with my baby and stuck without enough milk for him. Everyone kept saying 'get out and see your NCT people' 'join a baby group' etc. I just wanted to see my v close family, my husband, one or two friends."

I told her that I was very wary of other new mothers at that time, because I could not stand to hear their descriptions of it all as "a constant joy" and how in love with their child they were. I could not begin to relate. I thought it might be helpful for Sarah to hear this perspective as we tend not to realise other mums may be feeling this way.

"The recovery has been gradual and subtle, so I can't pinpoint turning points (apart from the drugs!) but I would say that my husband gave me some great advice. When I said 'I can't do it', he said 'you ARE doing it. You're keeping our baby clothed, fed, clean. That's a huge job and you're doing it'. He also, when I was stressing about not being adventurous enough and going on all sorts of trips with my baby, said 'do what you need to, when you want to' - basically don't feel pressured into doing any more than you feel able to do. I leant on him enormously, he came home early from work for weeks to help me - I remember in weeks three and four he'd get back every day and I'd be sitting there holding Joe and sobbing. I also got my mum down from Scotland for two extended stays and really leant on her too - including handing Joe over to her in the middle of the night once so I could just get a few hours sleep. Sleep makes SO much difference - sounds obvious - but so true. You can't underestimate what the lack of it will do to your state of mind. I did slowly start going out and about, at my own pace… I find it helps SO much because the days go really quick when you have stuff on. I do find I'm drawn to people who aren't all 'isn't it wonderful' - not to denigrate their experience but you have to be careful not to end up making comparisons. Your experience is just as valid. You are having a tough time - it's important to acknowledge it."

Sarah told me that she had hyperemesis gravidarum – the condition now better known because the Duchess of Cambridge has had it twice - which causes severe sickness and dehydration during pregnancy, sometimes requiring hospitalisation, throughout her whole pregnancy. Then, at the end of her pregnancy, she was diagnosed with obstetric cholestasis – a liver malfunction which can be fatal for the baby. She endured a 50 hour labour which she described as "traumatic… even thinking about [it] now makes me feel dark." What she struggled with after the birth was the desire to control everything and maintain her highly organised lifestyle. She found it difficult to adjust to new standards, and to the fact that she couldn't do very much having had an episiotomy so was physically limited, and she couldn't keep her home as organised as she had before. She describes the advent of the "blues" on day four along with her milk. But unlike the baby blues we all learn about in antenatal classes, these never went away. She started to experience invasive thoughts, and was so ashamed of this she didn't tell anyone for six weeks. Even when she did the Edinburgh Scale questions, she lied in her answers.

Things deteriorated further, and she moved back to her hometown to live with her parents. When she first emailed me, she said, "I wish I hadn't left it so long to be diagnosed, as I wouldn't be in this mess now. The worst of it has been me saying 'I just don't want to be here anymore', at which my family sat up and paid huge attention (after much sobbing)." She was then referred to the community mental health team, through whom she received CBT, along with anti-depressants and specialist help from a health visitor trained in mental health issues.

"At my lowest I have thought, 'No-one has had this like I have had this'; 'I am mad', 'I shouldn't be a mum, you will read about me in the Daily Mail for being the only woman on earth not wanting to be a mum'. I also blame myself for causing so much pain to my loved ones. Did you feel like that? I have felt so very down I can only describe it as a physical pain."

In my reply to Sarah, I told her that whilst she may have felt she didn't address the situation soon enough, in reality it was still very early and a very positive thing that she was already getting help. Interestingly for me, looking back, I also commented that I shared her dark feelings about remembering the labour (I don't now, these have faded). I do also think it's significant that she had serious medical complications. I have always thought that having pre-eclampsia had to somehow have contributed to my state of mind.

We also discussed the fact that recovery from depression does not always march forwards, that there are bad days, and that sometimes starting anti-depressants can make things initially feel worse, before they get better. We both were very fortunate to find Sertraline effective, although I know not everyone agrees with its efficacy. I was also struck by how positive Sarah already felt towards her son, as my own feelings had been more detached. I remembered that I would comment he was "cute" without feeling a great attachment. Reading the next line was very shocking to me, five years on from actually writing it: "But don't feel bad about the invasive thoughts - they really are so common. I've never told anyone this but I had them too."

And then:

"I did definitely find it an almost physical pain - like nausea or a huge weight on my body at times." What I find interesting looking back through our emails, is that there are some things I have completely forgotten (or blocked out). I have no memory of having invasive thoughts – but I know I would not have lied to Sarah about that. I don't even know what they would have been. I also have no memory of feeling physical pain as I describe in my email. I'm sitting in my garden in the September sun writing this, and I can hardly believe that something which happened only just over five years ago has receded to the point that parts of it (and quite traumatic parts by the sounds of it) have disappeared completely.

Later, Sarah sought reassurance that things would improve during a major dip. I was able to say that I had felt the same way. I told her:

"I was just asking my husband what I was like and he said I would say 'oh my god I'm never getting better' etc - then would have a 'good day' the very next day."

Sarah did a course of CBT and found it enormously helpful, so much so that two years later, when I had my second child, I pushed for it from the moment I was diagnosed with PND again – remembering how positive she had found the experience. Compare this line to her previous email:

"... suddenly I realised the other day I've had two bad days out of 20 (I've been making a note of good days). That is a better run than I've ever had since [her baby] was born so I know that I am getting better. My health visitor is really happy with the progress."

What I have found most PND sufferers have in common, in terms of finding a way out of the maze, is that we have all had something we have clung to which has helped, aside from professional help and medication, that is. So, for me, there were a couple of things: getting to know some like-minded mums in my local area – but through an online forum, not through the baby groups I was phobic of. Mums who, like me, didn't think the whole experience was a bed of roses, a magical time, or any of the other comments which seemed to fill articles in baby magazines. I also found something to do every week: I went along to the baby rhyme time at the local library I have already mentioned. I enjoyed the fact that this combined anonymity with getting out and being around people – may sound like an oxymoron, but it wasn't for me. But it's something different for everyone. For Sarah, rhyme time didn't suit her. I felt terrible because I encouraged her to go, and met her afterwards, only to find that she had felt the whole experience was embarrassing and nerve-wracking. It just wasn't for her. But she had a wonderful health visitor – who she mentions in her emails – who encouraged her to go to a local mums and babies group run by an NCT teacher who was well used to supporting mums who were struggling to cope. For Sarah, that group achieved what rhyme time did for me - just a short period each week when things didn't feel quite so bad.

The other thought that strikes me about reading these emails, is more a memory. When I had my second child I let Sarah know that I had PND again. She immediately, and with great presence of mind, reminded me of my very advice to her: that the bad days would make me feel like my recovery had stalled, but that I had to trust that it would get better. I don't think I would have accepted this from anyone else but because I knew I had advised her the same way in the past, and that she had recovered as I'd told her she would, I *knew* she was right.

I asked Sarah if she too would be prepared to reflect on that period, and share how she thinks of it now. She wrote back to me, saying:

"My expectations of motherhood were that I'd have a year off work to look after my baby. I didn't realise what 'looking after' really meant. I thought it meant soothing, feeding, changing nappies – without understanding the complex emotions I would feel as a result of this change in role. I had no idea of the relentless pace of motherhood, the effect that sleep depravity would have, how emotionally challenging it would be, how essentially, my whole existence that I knew previously (i.e. an independent person with only myself to look after) would disappear. My role as a mother is wonderful and amazing and I would never trade it with my life before children. However, it took me a long time to feel comfortable with the massive changes that come with motherhood and the sheer weight that comes with caring for something so precious and vulnerable."

Her main memory of her first labour was the length of time it took – she was shocked by this:

"For me it was 50 hours from my first contractions to birth. I don't think I slept a wink during the labour. It was absolutely exhausting. I was shocked by how medicalised it was. I had never suffered from any illness that has required hospitalisation before having children, so perhaps I was just naïve to the fact that labour can sometimes need medical intervention (something that certain childbirth/women's groups convince you is not a necessity), and if you are not used to hospitals and everything that you find in them - drips, heart monitors, stitches etc – this can actually seem very frightening. Particularly when your main concern is the health of your unborn child."

Her description of her first emotions on seeing her newborn child are really interesting (my own memory is extremely hazy on this, but I do not think I felt this way):

"I remember prior to the birth a few people had said that when the baby comes out it can look a little bit ugly and not to be surprised by that! So I was really shocked when I was presented with my child and he appeared to be the most beautiful thing I'd ever seen – it was like someone had flicked a switch inside me or turned a tap on, and I finally knew what unconditional love felt like."

However, the birth had left her deeply traumatised:

"I felt very uncomfortable when they lay him on me skin to skin, covered in blood... in hindsight I realise ... I was experiencing a mixture of feelings that I was unable to process i.e. a deep love combined with a feeling of anxiety and distress at what had just happened."

To compound matters, and in a sadly very familiar tale, Sarah's hospital experience was very unhappy – "abysmal", she says. In fact she thinks it played a big role in her developing PND. She had given birth to her son early evening, and made it onto the ward around 11pm that night.

"I felt an exhaustion I'd never known before and just wanted to sleep. I was still numb from the epidural and couldn't move or sit up properly, however, when my new baby cried (not having a clue what to do at this point!) he was simply placed under the crook of my arm and I was left to deal with it without any help at all. I was also very distressed that my husband had been asked to leave – he had been such an important support during the birth and in a way I needed him more after the birth – I felt incredibly vulnerable. But he was ushered out and told to come back the next day."

When I met Sarah for the first time, she told me about a shocking incident which happened the morning after her son was born. It has stayed with me because I think it truly is every mother's nightmare, and I feel incredibly sad for her that it happened.

"My son had to be taken away to a paediatric ward to have a few tests. When he was returned to me 20 minutes later (by this point I'd not slept for over 72 hours) they explained that he had been turned away from the paediatric ward as he didn't have any wrist or ankle ID bands on him – I was therefore asked to verify whether I believed they had my son in their arms so that they label him up correctly. The midwife in question even joked that she'd also misplaced another baby and she hoped that the child she was holding (i.e. my child) wasn't actually another child. This incident deeply affected my ability to bond with my baby from that point – when I went home I started comparing some photos that had been taken within an hour of his birth, with ones that had been taken the following day (after this event) to check whether they looked like the same child. Part of my recovery from PND involved writing to [the hospital's patient liaison service] about the incident and having it fully investigated. It was hence revealed that when such an incident occurs it is escalated to the matron and head of midwifery and an immediate investigation takes place in situ so that parents can be reassured. This did not happen and was never offered, and as such the hospital admitted a complete failure to adhere to policy and process. I received a formal apology from the hospital Chief Executive."

This must have been a deeply shocking experience. But, she says, she doesn't think it is policies which are to blame, but understaffing of post-natal (and labour) wards. She compares them to a "factory production line – unless something goes very wrong". Like many women, her mother was of a generation where she was kept in hospital for a week to recuperate from her birth and establish feeding. She therefore went home "well rested and emotionally well... There is something very wrong with a society that doesn't nurture new mothers both physically and emotionally."

She feels she was unprepared for how long the post-natal recovery would take: "I just needed to rest but was unable to sleep due to the anxiety I felt following on from the birth."

Sarah very quickly realised something was wrong. She would find herself at the kitchen sink, and suddenly realising that the hot water had run cold and she had lost half an hour standing there, reliving the birth. She told her midwife what was happening, who, after a few more visits, summoned the GP for a home visit. He prescribed her sleeping tablets. To his credit, he did spot the signs of PTSD straightaway, but said that the waiting list to be seen would be six months. He and Sarah's midwife disagreed about next steps – the midwife insistent that she be referred to the community mental health team to access help straight-away. The GP suggested that the case did not merit immediate treatment, as she was not showing signs of psychosis. Naturally, this tension served only to compound Sarah's feelings of confusion and vulnerability. Going to stay with her family was the first step. There, she received support from family, old friends, and a local midwife, who quickly directed her to the local GP. Here she received - at last - proper understanding of what she was going through, and was treated by professionals with good knowledge of perinatal mental health. Her story might have been an upward trajectory from here, but the couple made the fateful decision to return to their own home.

"I suddenly found myself isolated in our flat, without any family (or many friends). I felt terribly low and my feelings were compounded by my isolation. I'd also started to consider that having PND was something to be ashamed of – and though it had been suggested by most of the doctors and midwives as being something I possibly had or would be diagnosed with, I felt like I needed to go to great lengths to prove this was not the case. Essentially, it would prove I was a failure at being a Mum."

To prove she was on top of things, Sarah would clean the house obsessively ahead of visitors. She felt she was in some way balancing her feelings about the difficult birth and the lack of sleep by being incredibly organised at home and keeping the flat presentable. Of course now she acknowledges that in doing this she was exhausting herself still further. This, along with difficulties breast-feeding, combined to make her feel "demoralised, and like a complete failure".

"I remember telling people (before I was diagnosed with PND) that I just didn't feel right as it seemed as though someone had drugged me with a depressant. I knew that the labour had upset me but I also knew that it wasn't normal to feel the way I did to such an extent. I was surrounded by congratulations cards and bouquets of flowers, but my mood didn't reflect the way that a new mother probably should feel i.e. elation… I simply couldn't explain why I felt so sad all the time. I knew I loved my little boy but I felt so guilty that

I was a sad mother – I felt like I was letting him down before I'd even started to be his Mum."

That feeling of responsibility is one I recognise, and I'm sure many others will too. It can be very overwhelming, suddenly feeling the weight of that responsibility to your child. Sarah felt guilty about having had to ask her loved ones for help – she knew she was worrying them.

"Having depression changed my life and opened my eyes to what it feels like to be seriously ill. It was like I had become a shell, that nothing was working properly, and that there was no light at the end of the tunnel... I felt like even on a sunny day all I could experience was a feeling of the sun being behind the clouds – literally like I was wearing blue/grey tinted sunglasses all the time. I couldn't sleep even though I needed to desperately. I felt in a constant state of anxiety – so acute that it felt like every nerve ending in my body was constantly electrified."

Unable to relax, at its worst Sarah's anxiety left her unable to hold a conversation or concentrate on a TV programme. She describes a sensation of "constant weight" in her chest, and a sob in her throat. She also began to experience something that was very frightening for her:

"...I'd started to imagine awful things happening – I became scared of leaving the flat in case I fell down the stairs with the baby in my arms and he died. I didn't want to bath him in case he drowned – I'd literally imagine that happening and recoil, and think I was some kind of monster for having such horrible thoughts and therefore that I could never tell anyone how I felt."

When she lied to the health visitor at six weeks, answering the Edinburgh Scale questions, she says that she found the whole experience very intrusive, "having a complete stranger come into my house with a clipboard asking me very personal questions about how I felt. As such, I lied when giving the answers and my score came out fine – I officially didn't have PND and was well. The next day, realising what I'd done and that my safety net was gone – essentially, that no-one was looking out for me any more – I had a complete breakdown. I managed to call my Mum and tell her that really things were very bad, that I simply couldn't pretend any more, that things were not fine, and that I needed to come and stay and get help and a proper diagnosis. My boyfriend drove us all up the next day and a few days later I was properly diagnosed with PND by a very sensitive and caring Health Visitor who didn't have a clipboard in her hand and didn't need a form or tickboxes to annotate when talking to me. She didn't make me feel like a lab rat but like a human being. She kindly explained that the horrible visions I'd been having were called intrusive thoughts – it was such a relief to know that they had a name and that I wasn't the only person who'd experienced this before."

By this stage, Sarah was very unwell, but in a way she feels that this allowed her to finally access the health care she had needed from the start. She was routed to community mental health support, referred for CBT, and put on anti-depressants. She is clear that there was no instant fix. But simply being diagnosed was a relief:

"I was actually ill, I could stop pretending to people – I could let myself be helped. I wasn't struggling because I was an inadequate mother – I was struggling because I was very unwell, and when I was better, I'd be able to take on my new role as Mum."

Sarah went on to have a daughter a few years later. We had discussed what it would be like having another child given our experience first time around, and she was a great support to me when I succumbed to PND a second time. So when she went on to have her little girl, I was concerned about whether she too would become ill again. She admits she was anxious about developing PND again, but says that the community midwife team whose care she was under was very supportive.

"My second labour was once again medicalised due to a gestational liver condition I had developed, however, I didn't have the same feeling of fear that I'd had the first time around. When the baby was born my midwife found me a private room so that I could get some sleep that I so desperately needed and was deprived of the first time around. Instead of being lectured to about the benefits of breast-feeding, I was allowed to jointly breast- and bottle-feed my daughter in hospital without quibble, so that I could rest. My husband was also allowed to stay overnight with me (on a beach lilo that my midwife had kindly brought in for him!). When I was released from hospital I was given the option of staying longer if I wished (in the private room) and was also given proper medication for my stitches so I wasn't in the pain I had been previously.

As I had a specialist midwife I had continuity of care and knew that my hand was being held – that I had someone looking out for me, who knew me well enough to know if I was becoming unwell. She visited me at home for a few weeks after birth, ensuring that myself and my baby and my husband were all well. I'd lost a lot of weight due to the morning sickness, and was quite weak, but my midwife nurtured me and gave me the confidence that I'd get better and that she was on my side. It was such a stark contrast to my previous experience. All of this, combined with the love of my family and friends, meant that I had a truly joyful post-natal period the second time around."

Things threatened to derail around three months in, when her partner lost his job, and her only grandparent died. She began feeling anxious again, which had a physical manifestation (Irritable Bowel Syndrome). However, she was very self-aware this time. She knew that her anxiety was disproportionate, and she quickly sought a referral for CBT from her GP. Fortunately, she was seen within a few weeks. "Though I didn't feel depressed, and the anxiety wasn't on the same scale as it had been previously, I knew from my first experience that it was best to nip such symptoms in the bud early on – and as such I didn't become ill, and my anxiety dissipated very quickly."

The logistical difficulties of having two children are well documented but, interestingly to me, the people I have spoken to whilst writing this book have widely varying experiences of this. Some feel it's a case of 'better the devil you know' – they already know what they are doing, it's just one more, and, apart from the unavoidable sleep deprivation, they adjust relatively smoothly. I would say Sarah falls into that category. "I have a 2.5 year age gap between children and though juggling two children is hectic, it was probably the easiest part of my motherhood experience as I was already 'doing' all the mum stuff anyway so to do it for a second wasn't as big a shock as it had been first time around."

Since the birth of her second child, she has moved to another area – away from the specialist midwife support she received during that pregnancy and birth. She feels it's unlikely she could access similar support in her new area, and that is a factor in thinking about having further children.

Some women, myself included, who have had PND can be almost too open about the hard bits around motherhood, in an effort to prepare people. Sarah takes a more diplomatic approach:

"I never share my story with anyone expecting a child… I wouldn't want to worry any expectant mums. I do confess that it is very hard work having a new baby but most importantly I tell them that in the end being a mum is a life-changingly joyous experience – because it is."

However, her experience has left her with a strong desire to help others going through what she did. She has become a volunteer through the Association for Post Natal Illness (APNI) to provide support to women going through similar experiences. She comments that being connected to another mum who had had PND (me!) was "invaluable, and I believe is an essential treatment that should be offered to all mums with PND." To the mothers she has helped via APNI, she has said:

"You will get better… keep seeing your doctor/health visitor/counsellor." She is very keen to add that PND is something that can of course only be diagnosed by a health professional, and that "it is really important that families of new mothers who are struggling understand that. They may think they are being helpful by providing their own diagnosis and opinions, but really this is an illness like any other, and the only way to recover is to get a proper diagnosis and a proper plan for recovery from a clinical expert."

The experience of PND stays with her. "It has completely changed my life, mostly for the better. I never take health for granted any more. Though I say the experience has improved my life, I would never want it repeated. Having a nervous breakdown is a life catastrophe… it ripped me apart and was deeply upsetting for my family. However, it does mean that I have an understanding of mental health that I didn't have before and it has given me a respect for mental health that I think is so very important, particularly in my role as a Mum. My key goal as a Mum is to bring up two children who are healthy and happy."

Reflecting on her experience, she believes two things which contributed to her illness have not yet improved, one being disconnected health services – it should not have taken as long as it did for her to receive a diagnosis, and support. Having sought treatment in two different cities, she also became aware of the inconsistencies between different places: "It is desperately sad that the likelihood of a mother's recovery is dependent on where they live…"

Secondly, she feels strongly that our society doesn't nurture new mothers enough. It "expects them to be out and about putting on a brave face within a day of their labour." As I write this, the image of the Duchess of Cambridge, ten hours after giving birth to her second child, standing on the hospital steps with her baby, a blow-dry, heels and a shift dress is splashed across the front of every newspaper. Of course, it's a good thing if everything has gone well to move around, and if you really can do all those things well, why not? - but I see Sarah's point. Not everyone has had a trauma-free birth. Not everyone feels like smiling. She says, "Yes some mums are able to do that, but you never know what their back story is – perhaps they had a really easy labour and birth. I just wish women were more honest about it all and it was a more accepted conversation piece rather than a given that having children is a part of a woman's life much like buying your first home and getting a promotion. It is far more important than either of these things and should not be treated in the same way."

Trauma
Tabitha's story

Tabitha has three children, two girls and a boy. She sums up an experience many first-time parents can probably relate to, when she thinks back to what she thought it would be like having a baby: "I thought it would be like looking after a cat. I didn't buy any cat care books when I got a cat, but managed fine. However, when my daughter, now 10, arrived, it was a shock as I had no idea how to look after her… she did unpredictable things (I couldn't put her down without her yelling!). I remember panic-buying baby books from Amazon and trying to cram while breastfeeding (which was very hard)."

I can completely relate to this (right down to the panic Amazon spree). I remember the feeling of total bewilderment when I realised Joe wasn't going to just lie around in a Moses basket all day. Tabitha also says, "I think I assumed mothering was common sense and would come naturally." How many times did we all hear the irritating "Mama knows best" maxim first time round? "Go with your instinct" is great advice *if* you actually have the instincts.

Our relationships with our own mothers, and with existing and new friends – particularly female – come into a new focus after motherhood. Tabitha, like many women I know, was fortunate to have a good and supportive NCT group who she credits with keeping her sane. Her mother was supportive too and visited regularly. However, like my own mother, Tabitha's mum had found breast-feeding very easy. I remember finding this frustrating, although my mum quickly saw how much I was genuinely struggling with Joe. I've heard this from other new mums, and wonder if it's a generational thing. Do our mothers look back with rose-tinted glasses (the way we looked forward once)? Breast-feeding may be 'natural' but, as a friend once noted to me, after I'd mastered it second time around but not found it to be the panacea I'd expected, "natural doesn't mean easy."

Tabitha is very honest about breast-feeding. "I hated it. I always felt guilty that I drank too much wine! And I often found it agonisingly painful."

Another thing which anecdotally many of my mum's generation seem to do is to claim we were all sleeping through almost immediately. Can this really be true?! Perhaps the fact baby monitors hadn't been invented had more to do with it... or again, perhaps it's the same instinct which prompts them to tell us labour wasn't too bad.

Tabitha thinks she probably had depression after her first child, but it was not diagnosed. The birth itself she describes as fine. The next day she said she would happily do it again. But she says: "She didn't look like I had expected her to look, I didn't know what to say to her, and she felt quite alien. It took a while to bond, poor love. I remember waking up in the night to find her awake and quietly staring at me, and it totally freaked me out! I would like to go back and do it differently... It took me a long time to get used to being a mother. I felt my life had been hijacked. I remember saying goodbye to my husband in the morning and feeling utter despair about the ten hours till he got home and I could put my daughter to bed!! I hated all the unscheduled time. I felt invisible. I hated being on call night and day. But then I hated going back to work too, and felt really guilty and knackered."

Tabitha's second labour was traumatic. "I had a placental abruption and my waters were eventually broken in hospital to induce labour." Her baby's heart rate was erratic, and at one point a monitor attached to her head wasn't turned on, so Tabitha thought her baby had died. "She was born by ventouse delivery without pain relief and the pain was extraordinary. I felt like my body was being ripped apart. I guess it was. I had muscular pain so bad from bracing my body against the floor in labour that I needed painkillers for several weeks afterwards." Tabitha's daughter has a disability, which she strongly believes was caused by her pre-natal care. As a result, Tabitha has PTSD, particularly around the subject of midwives – she can hardly bear to say the word. "My heart rate increases if I even hear it or read it." Sadly her care did not immediately improve after the birth either. She had to ask not to be seen by one particular health visitor after she had told Tabitha a story about a baby dying after spending time in the Neonatal Intensive Care Unit (NICU). This was a few days after her baby had come home from NICU, after three weeks on a ventilator, full of anticonvulsants.

As a consequence of that hugely distressing experience, Tabitha opted for an elective C-section with her third child – but had to argue strongly for it.

Tabitha also had depression after her second child, due to the traumatic circumstances of her birth: "I was watching her all the time to see if she was fitting, I had no idea how her development would pan out, and I was very depressed for a while. I would go as far as saying I felt suicidal at times. I couldn't eat, I lost lots of weight, and I used to imagine just driving the car off the road. I just wanted to sleep, all the time. I had to act a bit normal for my older daughter's sake but used to cry a lot. I remember her saying 'why is mummy crying again?' and it broke my heart." Things got better by the time her second child was about four months old.

Interestingly, when Tabitha had her third child, she didn't get depressed. She describes life as "utterly chaotic...

I could hardly keep the show on the road. But I really enjoyed looking after him. Just for some reason it all clicked into place. If he cried, I didn't take it personally, I could just patiently absorb his upset without getting stressed myself, or feeling inadequate. When (my first) cried I remember putting her in her basket and getting into bed and crying too!"

The big question for a lot of parents who have been affected by PND is, would you do it again? For my part, it's a question we have chewed over often, sometimes with different conclusions. In Tabitha's case, in common I suspect with many mothers, she says that despite feeling broody when she sees babies, she loves her new-found freedom. She freely admits she found playing with (small) children boring. Now, a bit older, they are more like little companions. "They are funny, they say such funny things." She also reflects that in some ways it got easier with each child. "I need structure, I have a very strong need to be in control and have plans, schedules and to do lists. New (first) babies involve a lot of free-form floating through the days (and nights) and that is not me at all."

Anxiety
Lauren's story

Something which several of the professionals I spoke to, and Ruth at Bluebell Care, commented on was the high incidence of anxiety rather than depression in new mothers. I spoke to Lauren who went through this when her first son was born in 2010. She went into motherhood with a fairly realistic view (unlike many women), saying "I was expecting it to be hard and it was! Never felt such extreme emotions – joy but also helplessness and at times crippling anxiety." She was well supported by family but they lived at least two hours away, so though they visited when they could, they couldn't be there all the time.

She tells me that her first son was born two weeks early. She had barely started her maternity leave, and in fact was visiting family at the time – so ended up not having him in the hospital she had planned to be in. Not surprisingly, she remembers feeling very unprepared. I feel myself that not having any maternity leave was a factor in my depression. There was no demarcation and no rest between a hectic job and the new baby explosion.

Lauren's birth itself was straightforward, but she says the hospital was "awful". She was left on her own on a ward and never examined – in fact told to keep the noise down by midwives who did not realise she was in active labour until 30 minutes before she gave birth. Nevertheless, she felt she bonded with her son immediately, and felt "elated". Her post-natal stay was not great. She received no help with breast-feeding, and feels part of the problem was the midwife took her baby away so she could rest, and gave him a bottle. I told her that I felt the opposite: that if the (overstretched) midwives had been able to do that when Joe was born, I may have caught up on some sleep, and not got into the downward spiral of exhaustion. But we had different situations and different needs, and if anything these two stories surely tell us that what matters is not so much what the staff do in a particular situation, but whether they are listening to the patient and providing true "patient-led" care. Happily, when she had her second son four years later she was in a different hospital, was well supported and is still breast-feeding him now.

After her first son, her husband had started a new job and was unable to take leave. She says those first few weeks were a blur. She began quite early on to feel anxious about driving, her fear being she would crash and hurt her baby. This was a vicious circle: where she lived, she was ten miles away from her NCT friends, so to see them she needed to drive - but felt unable to, so would miss the meet ups, leaving her feeling worse, and isolated. Then there was a period of heavy snow and she barely left the house for a month. Her husband's new job was a two hour commute away, meaning he was away for long days, and she was also the one getting up in the night. The resulting exhaustion left her feeling she could not cope.

The background to Lauren's anxiety issues starts before pregnancy. She was already receiving CBT, which continued after she had her son. Her therapist eventually suggested she go on an anti-depressant called citalopram, when her son was six months old. Up until then, she says she "consciously hid (the depression) as I felt that I would be a failure if I went on anti-depressants. I didn't connect my anxiety with PND." In hindsight, she feels she waited far too long to start them. "However I felt so much better once I started taking them that I realised how down I had been. CBT was useful, but I needed a leg-up with the drugs to get me to a point where I could put the CBT techniques into practice." She also makes a very interesting point which I think is very much of its time. She says that it may sound ridiculous but having the use of an iPad second time around made her feel less isolated. She could access information about any worries or problems straightaway, internet forums provided reassurance that other people were having the same problems, and social media provided a connection to the outside world during marathon cluster feeds. I definitely noticed the difference after my second, when I had a smartphone and I could stay connected even when it felt as if I was living on a completely different timeline to the rest of the world. Despite Lauren's struggle with anxiety, she does reflect that she enjoyed the break from work. It gave her the chance to spend time in her home town (she commuted to work so up until now had not spent much time there), and made a life for herself there. She made good friends and says today she feels very happy. "I have got to grips with my anxiety issues, so I'm a lot happier." Her second birth felt better, she took more time off before it, and overall life with her second child has felt smoother. She has kept on the childcare she had in place when she was in work, helped by childcare vouchers, and has help from family, so juggling the two children has not felt overwhelming. The age gap is four years, and she says it took her two years to be able to think about having another after her first was born.

She says being a mother is "the most terrifying, but most rewarding thing you'll ever do. It will change your life forever for the better. It will get easier, but in the meantime take any help you can with both hands." She adds, "I wish I had asked for help sooner."

10

Coping with PND second time around

I'm quite interested in how those with repeated experiences of PND find the second time around – are there differences? Are we better equipped, as I had hoped and assumed from my first birth to my second? It wasn't a straightforward answer in my own case.

Initially, after Ted was born, I felt fine – which was different to my experience with Joe, when I had felt consumed by unhappiness after the first night. When Ted was ten days old, I wrote to a friend who had also had PND after her first:

"It is totally mad with two, but also quite lovely. Am a bit nervous about coping when Ben is back at work... but my mum is coming down for a few days to help ease the transition. I think though that even when things seem tough - and have def had some of those dark cloud moments which you probably remember - at least I kind of know what I'm dealing with, so am fully prepared to go for the drugs/counselling if I feel I need it, though so far think am fine as long as I get some sleep/food!"

And yet things changed quite soon after this, as later emails show, perhaps down to the onset of Ted's reflux I described earlier. Like many mums when dads first go back after paternity leave, I had that terrible sense of panic – how would I cope? But I knew that this was more than just natural nervousness, I felt absolutely beside myself with fear.

To any enquirers, I would say jokingly, oh it's like a relay with two. If it's not one, it's the other kicking off, and sometimes both, just for bonus fun. But beneath that appearance of organised chaos, I actually felt truly chaotic. On the way to a party at Joe's nursery, with Ted in the sling, I tripped on some wet leaves and fell. I was fairly sure Ted hadn't been hurt but did wonder if his head was ok, where it was poking out of the top of the sling. I remember walking into Joe's nursery and asking the nursery workers and other mums what to do. I felt as though I had lost all sense of proportion and normality, as if I just didn't know what the right thing to do was any more. Where were those instincts again? Could someone just tell me what to do?

By the time Ted was six weeks old, I wrote a message to an NCT friend:

"Ted is six weeks and we're not as settled as I'd hoped to be by now - he started off really chilled out but then got reflux like Joe, only much worse. Doesn't sleep much at all, and is v v unsettled and sore a lot of the time. Makes the adjustment to 2 all the harder! We saw a specialist on Weds who gave us some serious drugs for it plus prescribed special dairy-free formula as it might be cow's milk protein allergy. Just hope it sorts itself soon. Was so hoping for an easy baby this time! But know I was lucky at least with Joe's sleep so perhaps am owed a bad sleeper.

Ted's birth was not great. I had to be transferred in from home birth and felt quite upset afterwards, I begged for an epidural right at the end (fully dilated - should have known better really but was past reason) - and then it didn't work! Argh. So [I] have ended up with post-natal depression again, but have drugs for it and things are slowly improving."

At this point, the nights were terrible. In a message to Ben, I said something which reminds me very much of how I felt about accepting help first time round too:

"Mum saying she'll do tonight... Sigh, know what you mean re help but also feel we do have to manage on our own eventually. Ted following usual pattern today despite our best efforts. Last night was so awful."

What I meant was that I felt I had to learn how to handle it, so what was the point of accepting any help? Of course in my non-PND state I can see how illogical this was. But I felt it very keenly. I had to prove to myself I could do it. This was probably linked to those awful first days when Ben went back to work both times. I can see from emails, and remember it well too, that a close friend tried admirably hard to get me to leave both boys with her (and her one year old) so I could have a haircut. I just couldn't allow myself to do it. I was so worried that Joe would play up for her. I knew I wouldn't enjoy the time out because I would be too anxious. Of course this mean I denied myself any respite, because the list of people I would allow to have both boys was very short. In fact, I think that perhaps the first time I let it happen was my first CBT session, when Ben took time off work to have the boys for two hours. I was gratified when he called me after and said, "It's hard work this, isn't it?" I had been very nervous when my new therapist rang me to introduce herself, and made it clear that if at all possible I would need to go to sessions alone – i.e. find childcare for Ted. Fortunately he wasn't exclusively breast-feeding so this wasn't completely impossible, but it was still a hurdle to get over. Whilst not an option for everyone, – and I realise how fortunate I was to be able to go alone – having been to therapy sessions both on my own and on occasion with a baby, I can see how much difference it makes. For me, I found it very hard to talk about how sad I felt, with my baby in my lap. I found I did instinctively soften what I had to say, even if the baby was just a few weeks old. It is just too jarring an image, and some of my hardest memories are the times when things were so bad I would be sobbing and explaining how miserable I felt, whilst holding my baby. Although recently I talked to a therapist who advocates mums bringing their baby to sessions, she gave me a different perspective.

Kathy's story

Kathy has two children, both of which were home births. She had PND after both. In contrast to some of the women I've spoken to, Kathy didn't have a rose-tinted view of motherhood before she had her own children.

"My expectations were quite limited. I was never a person who was certain I wanted children and I didn't have a particularly positive view of what it would be like, but nor did I expect it to be very negative. I was the youngest child in my family and rarely around children younger than me and never really around babies. So it was a very new experience. Our choice to start trying to have a family was rather based on the fact it seemed like the thing to do next."

In common with many affected by PND though, she found the experience of motherhood when it came profoundly shocking:

"The reality of motherhood was a massive smack in the face - physically, mentally, socially, everything-ally. The reality is very, very tough, or it was for me, and I had no expectation that I would find it so very hard."

This was despite what Kathy describes as "excellent midwives": "This is probably the only part of my experience that I would wish other people to have. The benefit of a [community] midwife practice is so valuable - a named midwife who goes through your pregnancy with you and delivers your baby (if they are working at that time), who stays with you whether you have your baby at home or in hospital and in my case kept coming to see me for ten days after the birth. Amazing support."

She did not find the visitors she came into contact with particularly effective, and found breastfeeding support to be poor, other than one person who was based at the local hospital and was "the only person… who seemed to be able to understand my very complicated breastfeeding problems."

I was interested to hear Kathy's take on the role a partner should play in supporting a mother, particularly one with PND – it chimed with my own thinking on this sometimes tense issue. People sometimes tell me I'm lucky to have Ben, given how supportive he has been. I feel lucky to have Ben, it's true. But I don't believe that equality should be down to luck. She agrees:

"My partner has always tried very very hard to support me and believes in equal parenting, so in many ways his support was brilliant… I refuse to be grateful for equality!"

Kathy's partner took his two weeks of paternity leave as well as an additional week of annual leave – three weeks in total – after both her births. "This seemed incredibly short. The day he was due to go back to work after my first child I remember being horrified that I had to cope alone."

She also hits on something which I think many PND

sufferers can related to: "Not to mention I am *useless* at asking for help. Really bad at it."

Kathy describes her first birth as "Uncertain and scary. I had my birth at home and it was quite long and hard. I found the idea that I was to spend so much of my labour on my own surprising and I wish that was more clear to women - whether they are at home or in hospital. Generally though my birth, compared to many people, was without major incident, without drugs, but with some tearing. The midwives went home and I went to bed. That was both wonderful and terrifying."

Despite this ostensibly good start, she describes feeling traumatised in the months afterwards, though she thinks this could have been down to ill health. When she discusses her second labour, which she found easier than the first, she comments that labour is "the only bit of babies I'm good at." In contrast, she found maternity leave both times "a very miserable experience, I found very little joy in my babies." This was because she had endless health problems, which led to PND. Her first child did not sleep well, and the exhaustion combined with illness left her very low. "It was hard to adore the child whose arrival had coincided with all my pain." Despite this, she does not feel there was a lack of bonding. And with her second, she says it was "easier to separate the bad experience from him, and I rather doted on him." She wrote to me though that it is only with some recent therapy that she has "managed to achieve a better state of mind about spending time alone with my children - which looks pretty bad now I see it written down."

Challenging the popular thinking that PND only sets in two weeks after birth, if not later, Kathy, just like I did, found things went wrong far earlier:

"With both my children everything went wrong on day three after the birth. When my milk came in I was then in a whole world of pain. Breast-feeding became a feat of endurance and I would sit in bed at night crying every time I had to do a feed because my nipples were completely raw - this happened very quickly with both babies. I had a terrible oversupply of milk so I was getting mastitis regularly - with the second baby it was within the first two weeks (and I had mastitis four times in the first three months). With my first baby I didn't go outside for quite a long time and I felt completely exhausted right after the birth, I was in a total haze. Coping with the health problems I was having took up my energy. With the second birth it was much easier and for the first two days I felt quite good, but on day three it all went wrong again."

Like so many others, Kathy did not receive a formal diagnosis of PND initially, which she describes as "worrying, as I think it was pretty obvious - I remember sitting in front of a GP crying about my breast-feeding problems and she basically told me there was nothing she could do. It felt like I was wading through mud, like my brain was working in slow motion, I couldn't do simple tasks easily, I felt very lethargic. I wanted to cry most of the time. I slept badly. I saw everything negatively. I was concerned about how I could bring children into such an awful world. I felt relentlessly defeated. I wanted to be dead - I didn't want to kill myself, but I felt very much that being dead would be better than being alive."

Kathy experienced ongoing stomach pains, which a gastroenterologist eventually diagnosed as stress related. This led to a referral to the local psychological services, including a group CBT course and a sleep workshop – the latter she describes as "one of the most useful courses I've ever done in my life." Follow-up sessions ensued and, as her first child got older, the depression did not go away – so she referred herself back for further therapy, and did a one-to-one CBT course.

Incredibly, no health professional picked up on her PND second time around either. Her midwife noted that she was at greater risk given she had had it first time around. She remembers going to her GP when her second baby was two months old. She was feeling "completely broken about breast-feeding" and begged the doctor for tablets to cut off her milk supply. She was prescribed them but did not take them, which she feels in hindsight was a terrible mistake. Later, she was given beta blockers, which were not sufficient, and then started on an anti-depressant called Citalopram which, she says,

"… improved everything massively, I wished I had taken it years ago. However when my son was about three [years] I started to dip again quite badly so I asked to get further one-to-one counselling. NHS response was so slow that I eventually went privately because I was desperate. I had a very productive and expensive course of sessions which were also CBT based but much more in-depth, and that has been hugely beneficial for me. I am currently in a position where I feel I might start reducing the dosage of my anti-depressant."

Considering what it was she found hardest, Kathy says that the "hard physical work was relentless yet at the same time it was incredibly boring." On top of that she was interminably ill and tired. She says she felt very lonely. She did not enjoy being on her own with her baby, and she envied her partner having an escape in work.

"I was so miserable and too ill and tired to drag myself out to get some stimulation by seeing friends in the evenings - I resented my friends for not seeing how unhappy I was - but

I didn't really tell them. I also felt very wary of spending money, which made the days harder. I missed the stimulation of work very much. I hated being trapped in one small town all the time - if I got to go somewhere on my own I felt completely elated - even if it was just a short trip on the bus."

Kathy cites the lack of stimulation as having a big effect on her state of mind: "I was so fed up of not having an interesting conversation all day – not only that, I felt I didn't have much of interest to say because my day involved only mundane chores." But there was also an unwelcome change in status:

"Something else that drove me mad was the way my position as a woman was suddenly completely changed. I had always lived an equal life with my partner and suddenly I felt that because I was a woman my life had changed beyond recognition. Men seemed to carry on with their lives as if little had changed after babies were born, while I felt my position in life was totally changed, my career was dying and I was fading away. It made me walk around in a constant rage. I was very angry."

Although her second labour felt easier, she thinks that PND second time around was possibly worse. She suggests that mothers with a history of PND should have extra support with subsequent children. "I feel I was left to crash and burn." With just under three years between the two children, Kathy, just like myself a few years later, found the juggling act of the baby and the toddler difficult: "I have a particularly bad memory of a picnic that went wrong and I was trying to get home, pushing the buggy down the street with the baby inside and the toddler on the buggy board - all three of us were crying."

Hearing this anecdote, I had a flashback of a similar scene from that stage in my own life. I recall arguing with a pharmacist in a supermarket about a prescription for dairy-free formula which I desperately needed for my younger son, then a baby, who was screaming with hunger. Meanwhile two-year-old Joe had quite literally kicked off, and was kicking his shoes all the way down the aisles, while I felt as though the eyes of South London's shoppers were upon me. I remember joining the boys in their bawling, to the horror of the pharmacist. I later posted this on Facebook and within minutes several people had replied "Been there." We really are not alone – but it certainly can feel like it.

Kathy says that despite the depression she feels the experience has changed her in positive ways: "I got perspective on life and what is important and what isn't. I learned how to say no to people, and after a long time, how to be kinder to myself. Also I would say you get absorbed into the community of an area in a way you never did before having kids, that's a really nice part."

For some women, it can seem as though PND was a temporary blip in their life, very unpleasant, but a discrete episode with a line under it. However Kathy has a different view, and one I can empathise with: "I am realistic about the fact it may now affect me for life. Accepting this is one of the recent hurdles I've had to get over."

As part of this, she is very definite about not having more children. She is clear that it would damage her mental health badly, and it is therefore out of the question. She still feels as though post-natal depression, or the experience of it, is part of her daily life. But she does now feel better than she has in a long time. She encourages others with PND to "be kind to yourself and ask for help without shame. I was brutal to myself. It never occurred to me that I was damaging myself when I persevered with breastfeeding (twice!) and struggling to cope on my own despite relentless bad health [and] depression. I should have stopped it. I wish I had had someone to say to me - give up, look after yourself, you are just as important as this baby." She adds: "Living away from your family makes having children much more difficult, think twice before moving away from friends and family, you need people around you."

Kathy says she feels bad as she's actually advised many people against having children, although she now feels differently. I think Ben and I did this too. And then felt a bit surprised and envious when some of those people went on to have children and seemed to sail through it! She comments, "now all my friends have small babies and my children are older I am able to tell them that it gets much better - that we have really happy times and that you do start to get your life back."

She has views on the policy around post natal care too:

"The government need to invest money in breast-feeding support, GPs need to have ANY training in breast-feeding - at the moment they don't, fathers need to get more paternity leave - and take it - I suggest a use it or lose it set amount. Also Surestart centres need funding, not shutting down - the more places parents have to go with their babies the better."

She emphasizes the importance of sharing the load, too, for those in relationships. "I'm fed up of seeing my friends slaving looking after their babies while their partners sleep in the spare room. Men should be splitting childcare equally. Recently I have changed from part-time work to full-time while my partner has now gone down to three days. This has helped my sense of self enormously. I recommend it to everyone."

11

The Late Visitor

Lucy's story

Lucy has one child, and returned to work six months after having her son. She explains to me that she tried for many years to get pregnant, so it was "a very nice surprise" when she found out she was pregnant. She had very little real expectations of motherhood. Lucy is refreshingly honest about the experience of pregnancy, which so often we are told is a time when we will be glowing with health and happiness. "I hated pregnancy and the limitations my body placed on me by this *thing* growing inside me like a parasite. (That sounds rather harsh, but I did feel completely taken over by my baby by the end)."

By contrast, Lucy describes the birth of her son as "pretty bloody amazing… it's probably one of the things I'm proudest of." From her description, Lucy had a dream homebirth. She was in her son's bedroom, with a close friend and her husband. Labour was relatively short, she spent time singing and even doing yoga. There was some yelling but "overall it was fabulous." As a result, Lucy suggests she had more emotional energy – not having had a long drawn out labour as so many first time mothers do – and this may have helped with early bonding.

So birth was straightforward, and she bounced straight back to life after, but thinks she did so perhaps too quickly. She was taken aback by the sheer array of decisions to be made. "Should I feed my baby now? Should we go out now? Should I change his nappy now or risk going out? How do I *be* a mother?" She describes standing in a queue at the pharmacy just two days after the birth, waiting for antibiotics to treat a tear infection she had contracted. She then spent a horrific night vomiting, shaking, having diahorrhea and being terrified about going to the toilet because of the pain she was anticipating. "That was definitely the low point." She comments that she didn't share a lot of her feelings at the time.

A few months in, she found she really enjoyed being on maternity leave – being her own boss, able to organise her day and life as she liked. She set herself a baseline: "as long as the same number of humans (and animals) are alive at the end of the day as at the beginning, and everyone's had some food and some rest, we've done well", which became her mantra for a while. It also sounds as though Lucy handled the sleep deprivation really well. The fact that her son loved a routine and liked to nap in his cot, meant she was at home for a big chunk of each afternoon. This could have been restrictive, but she remembers watching a lot of sport on TV and making a local friend who she did craft/ creative activities with while the babies played. At this point of reading Lucy's story, I felt slightly in awe, the idea of doing anything remotely creative beyond putting on makeup would have been completely exotic to me at this stage.

Lucy is one of the women I spoke to who, like myself, had a history of depression, which meant she had longer midwifery care than normal. She notes though that in her case she didn't feel that afforded her much support. Instead she looked to her sister, who had her second child at a similar time, and NCT friends as well as friends made in the local community.

Despite the very positive birth Lucy describes, and the way in which she bounced straight back, she does say that she didn't necessarily bond immediately with her son. But as he grew, and she got more back (a term I hear a lot from new mums), "in terms of eye contact, smiles, laughs, movement", she felt her love grew.

And then her story takes a new turn. "I think depression really hit me about six months after returning to work." She returned to work when her son was eight months old. Her partner took some unpaid leave to help with the transition, which she says worked really well. But she was working full time, in an extremely demanding job, coping with the pressure of a nursery pick-up looming over her towards the end of each day. She says that looking back she can see that she was not adequately supported in her job – and felt unable to ask for help. In the end, a nervous breakdown at work resulted in her being signed off for a few months. Now, several years on, Lucy comes across as someone who has a handle on her depression, but perhaps sees it as part of her life: "although the depression has and does recur I am now more aware of the signs and better able to do self-care in those situations. I also have an extremely supportive GP and have had extensive counselling (not available on the NHS unfortunately)."

Her experience has made her determined to help others in the same boat – returning to work after maternity leave and potentially struggling - or who have partners in the same situation. She advises friends on practical matters – little things like remember to buy lots of bin liners, loo rolls and paracetamol. Having experienced a tear during her own birth, she emphasises how important it is to be prepared for that eventuality. But she also says to friends, "visitors can be exhausting. Everyone wants to see the baby and have a cuddle, but often those are the times when you may want to be catching up on sleep, or just resting. It may help to 'bunch' visitors together into daytime and evening... or simply text everyone and say you'll be in touch once things have calmed down and keep visitors to close friends and immediate family only. Don't be afraid to cancel on people if you just don't feel up to it. Schedule some time or days when you and your partner have some time to revel in your baby in peace." If, like me, that's less revelling and more just trying to get to grips with what has happened in your life, that suggestion still stands.

12

The Professionals

I count myself among the well-meaning women, ex PND sufferers, who want to help mothers going through the same thing. But what I've learnt through writing this book is just how nuanced the situation can be. It was incredibly helpful to me to have someone – Liz – who provided peer support at a time when I needed it most. But, crucially, I was also being seen by my GP, a counsellor, and I was on medication. Provision in mental healthcare can be patchy; I won't argue otherwise. But when I'm asked by a friend, as happens quite often, "I have a friend, and she thinks she has PND, what should I do?", the very first thing I always ask is "has she seen her GP?". And if she has, and that meeting was unfortunately not helpful, I would suggest asking to see a second, or a third doctor – change practices if that is what it takes. Or try a different route – perhaps through a midwife, Children's Centre or health visitor. There are lots of helpful things friends and family can do. There are also some very practical steps which local and national charities can help mothers take. But there is another very important group of people who help women through perinatal mental illness: the medical and mental health professionals.

The Counselling Psychologist

"Shame is very powerful: it stops people talking." I was talking to Dr Helena Belgrave, a chartered counselling psychologist with a perinatal specialism. She was telling me about the value of therapy: when people come to therapy and start to talk, they realise their situation is not necessarily as horrendous or as shameful as they thought, they can start to feel "normal".

I had wanted to find out more about why people develop PND, and the part therapy can play in how they help themselves. Dr Belgrave works both in the NHS and in private practice, treating men and women with a range of mental health issues, but her particular area of expertise is perinatal mental wellbeing. It was many years after completing her undergraduate degree in psychology that she hit on the realisation that psychotherapy was her vocation. She trained in counselling psychology, which is both psychotherapy and psychological research training, and, from what she told me, the psychologist in her complements her psychotherapy training very well. I was interested to know why she chose perinatal mental health as a specialism. Dr Belgrave has two children of her own, and tells me that she had just had her first when she took on her first placement during her counselling psychology training. This was working as part of a psychiatrist's team, the specialism of which was perinatal mental health. It marked the start of her interest in specialising in the area. Now Dr Belgrave sees mothers and expectant mothers individually in both the NHS and privately, but also facilitates a group discussion at a pilates class for new mothers, and is hoping to expand into workshops.

Dr Belgrave explained that she works integratively, utilising theory and technique from existential, psychodynamic and person-centred approaches. However, in her perinatal work, the psychodynamic approach stands out as the most relevant due to its focus on relationship dynamics between the mother and baby, and on attachment, in this case, the type of attachment style that develops between the mother and baby. When we met up to discuss her work, I asked her to tell me more about the psychodynamic approach. She said that Freud's defence mechanisms – repression, regression, projection, reaction formation and sublimation – are good examples of ways in which we handle anxiety and other distressing thoughts or feelings. Part of applying psychodynamic theory to her work involves looking with a client at how her past may be affecting her present. This often involves uncovering what may have happened in the past, especially around her upbringing, family dynamics and her relationship with her own mother, which may now be affecting her ability to manage motherhood. To my layman's ears this sounded diametrically opposed to the popular perception of the CBT approach, the therapy which is often most readily available on the NHS. Now, having spent time talking to Dr Belgrave and others in the field, I realise that a good CBT practitioner should be able to incorporate relevant issues from a client's history.

Dr Belgrave also emphasised that there is still a place for the existential and person-centred approaches in her perinatal work, as the bigger issues of freedom, responsibility and choice lend themselves well to process, as does empowering the new mother to feel confident in her new role.

I quizzed Dr Belgrave about *why* people get PND. I knew it was a slightly facile question, but I wanted to know if there were obvious causes. "There's no hard and fast cause," she confirmed. She explained that some people are more vulnerable, based on difficulties in their childhood. Perhaps they were abused or neglected, and/or they may have had difficult relationships with their parents. I wondered if some people may be pre-disposed to depression – something I've questioned about myself.

Dr Belgrave also discussed personality traits. For instance, if you are someone who needs a lot of control, you may struggle with the seismic shift in your life. However, some people just get it, and it is not really clear *why*, as there could be multiple reasons. The fact is, for many, parenthood is a shock. The baby is born, and suddenly parents wonder what they used to do with all their time, because now there is none. How you adapt to and accept your situation may well determine whether you fall prey to PND. But there is another, far less predictable element: hormones. Talking this through with Dr Belgrave, she suggested I talk to the consultant psychiatrist she worked for in her first placement, Dr Rebecca Moore at Mile End Hospital.

Dr Belgrave talked about how women need to accommodate our new role of being a mother. As we talked, I jotted down a phrase which came into my head - 'changing the pecking order'. It reminded me of that feeling when the babies were little: that I was no longer the director of my life. A friend of my mum's said to her, "I could run an organisation of hundreds of staff. But I couldn't run my baby."

With Dr Belgrave and later Dr Moore, I also discussed PTSD and its role in perinatal mental illness. Dr Belgrave explained to me that often women have certain expectations about their births – I think many of us can relate to this – and if the reality does not match those expectations, we can feel angry, upset or surprised about the outcome. However, if the birth is traumatic, such as an emergency caesarean, a near death experience, or some other kind of crisis, the mother may develop PTSD, as she tries to make sense of what has happened and come to terms with it. PTSD has a number of symptoms including flashbacks, such as Sarah has described.

I'm very interested in medication as a treatment for depression, particularly post-natal. I'm very biased too – I did use it twice, and it felt very much as though it worked. In fact when my younger son was around two, I went back on to Sertraline, having previously weaned myself off it, and I'm still on it today. I asked Dr Belgrave her take on medication for a woman with PND, as a therapist. She thinks that anti-depressants can help some and not others. As their goal is to lessen the feelings of depression and sometimes anxiety, this could help in a therapeutic setting, as the client may be able to engage more with the process. She said that, in her experience, often women with PND are suffering more with anxiety than depression, and that certain anti-depressants can be effective for treating this. I've been told by GPs that Sertraline is one of them.

Something I've encountered both with the women I've spoken to in the course of writing this book, and through stories told on social media and elsewhere, is the challenge many face in simply being diagnosed. Quite a few women admitted to me that they had lied during the infamous "Edinburgh Scale" questionnaire – the set of questions used by primary care professionals to assess a new mother's state of mind. I remember finding and completing this questionnaire myself online, then doing it with a doctor later. In my case, I didn't lie – I already knew things were bad and wanted to deal with them, but it's understandable that for many women, the truth is so frightening – and unknown – that they feel they can't admit it, even to themselves. Our greatest fear is that our child will be taken away from us. Dr Belgrave agreed that this can be a worry for new mums facing PND. She said that patients might tell themselves that they are ok and that they can cope – in fact, when I brought this up with Dr Moore, she said some patients convince themselves they have a physical problem, because that feels more acceptable. Both also agreed that PND in men is overlooked, but Dr Belgrave mentioned a figure to me which shocked me: that there is a 20% chance of a PND sufferer's partner developing depression[1]. She is particularly interested in how a new baby affects men, as "the dads have to share you: and your kids often take precedence". I thought how differently we had felt when each of our children arrived. After we had had Joe, amid the daily onslaught of new challenges Ben and I had never felt so united. It wasn't exactly me and him against the world – we didn't feel *against* our new son, but it was very much a sense that we were a team coping with a particularly challenging task. After Ted, it was very different. Maybe that's because I initially did breast-feed, though not for very long, and we did introduce the bottle almost immediately for some feeds. Certainly, because he had reflux which was far more severe than Joe's had been, he needed a lot of comfort, and I often co-slept with him. I was more confident this time, whereas first time around I had looked to Ben for advice and reassurance on everything. Slowly it began to feel as though Ted and I were in a little bubble, not Ben and I.

A lot of people – patients and professionals – have mentioned the postcode lottery of perinatal care. Certainly the women I talked to, who come from all over the country, have had vastly diverse experiences. I talked to Dr Belgrave about the National Institute for Health and Care Excellence

---

1 UK Medical Research Council and University College London, 2010

(NICE) Guidelines around antenatal and post-natal mental health, which were updated in December 2014. These recognise that while mental health problems are often treatable, many (which occur in the perinatal period) go "unrecognised and untreated". Importantly, they state that their recommendations are for women who are planning pregnancy, as well as pregnant women and mothers of infants up to the age of one. I immediately thought of Joanne (see Chapter 17) when I read this, and the impact her struggle to conceive had on her mental health, although in reality I suspect this category is about women who may have histories of mental health problems and are considering having a child.

The recommendations include a suggestion that during a woman's "booking in" appointment, or first primary care appointment of the pregnancy, healthcare professionals should "consider" asking about their state of mind. This includes using an abridged version of the General Anxiety Disorder questionnaire (GAD) often used by medical professionals, the longer version of which (GAD-7) I got to know very well when I was undergoing CBT. NICE Guidelines make a clear recommendation for "clinical networks", which when I met with Dr Rebecca Moore I learnt more about. These should provide "a specialist multidisciplinary perinatal service in each locality."

I hear a lot of different statistics over the prevalence of PND (and indeed antenatal depression - AND), but the ones NICE lay out are: "…around 12% of women experiencing depression and 13% experiencing anxiety at some point; many women will experience both." And beyond - "Depression and anxiety also affect 15-20% of women in the first year after childbirth."

A principle of care set out in the new version of the Guidelines instructs: "Acknowledge the woman's role in caring for her baby and support her to do this in a non-judgmental and compassionate way." Crucially, there is an emphasis on action being taken "in a timely manner", recognising the state a woman may be at in her pregnancy, or the age of her child if she has delivered. There are some quite specific guidelines on this, stating that when a woman with a known or suspected mental health problem is referred during pregnancy or after, they should be assessed for treatment within two weeks of referral, and receive psychological interventions (i.e. appointments with a therapist, whether one-to-one or within a group) within one month of initial assessment. This is actually a new detail in the updated Guidelines, but I was fortunate to receive support to a timetable that fairly closely resembled this, back in 2011, through the Maudsley Hospital.

And there is an understanding that mothers lie. "Recognise that women who have a mental health problem (or are worried that they might have) may be... unwilling to disclose or discuss their problem because of fear of stigma, negative perceptions of them as a mother or fear that their baby might be taken into care..."

There is a recommendation that women with a history of severe mental illness should be referred for secondary mental health support. And then a sentence which, while hardly news, is difficult reading for any PND sufferer: "Problems in the mother-baby relationship in the first year after childbirth may increase maternal mental health problems and are associated with a range of problems for the baby, including delayed cognitive and emotional development." Difficult to read it may be, but it also underlines why seeking help *early* is so important.

But of course, these are just guidelines and recommendations, as more than one professional has pointed out. My sample for this book is not particularly large but I've talked to people involved in lobbying for improved consistency and higher standards of perinatal mental healthcare and it's clear that the Guidelines are not being adhered to with any consistency. Dr Belgrave is among them: she feels strongly that perinatal care is very important, that care should start when the pregnancy starts, continuing after birth, so that parents are set on the right track. I have to agree that it seems a no-brainer: spend preventatively rather than skimp on the perinatal care and having to address problems in children further down the line.

What would Dr Belgrave's advice be to the women who do end up with PND?

"Don't suffer in silence – if you feel you are struggling to cope tell someone. It can be daunting, but empowering. Take it seriously – society may think that you need to be a 'supermom', but the reality is it can be hard work where some support may help you in both the short and the long-term."

The Consultant Perinatal Psychiatrist

After I left Mile End Hospital, where I went to interview Dr Rebecca Moore, a consultant perinatal psychiatrist who runs Tower Hamlets Perinatal Service, I called my mum: I was completely wired. I mean that in a positive sense, in that speaking to her had left me so enthused about her way of working, but there was an inevitable bittersweet edge: I wished I had received the level of care she outlined to me.

Dr Moore founded the Tower Hamlets Perinatal Service in 2008. Talking to her, I could see just how well women under her care must be looked after. She came across as modest on this point, and said that they simply adhere to the "gold standard" – and it's a standard I think most women whose stories appear here would love to be better acquainted with.

Dr Moore came to perinatal psychiatry fairly early in her career. She'd completed her medical degree, had a spell in A&E and then specialised in psychiatry. In one of her first jobs, she had a consultant who was very interested in perinatal psychiatry, this in the early days of work on perinatal mental health. She describes her then consultant as "a champion of women's health: really inspiring". A stint at Bethlem Mother and Baby Unit (MBU) followed–I had already had the good fortune to meet their inspiring staff, though not as a patient. After a year of research into PND, Dr Moore moved to Tower Hamlets and set up the perinatal service there. When I asked why it was that their standard of support was so high, she commented that "East London is very well resourced compared to a lot of areas in the country, although there is an increasing drive to address that inequality". She explained that the population in Tower Hamlets is young, with a high birth rate, and often larger than average sized families. There are clearly also areas of severe deprivation. "As a clinician it's a really interesting and exciting place to work: we see a lot of different clinical presentations." It is a transient area, with people arriving from around the world to settle there. "A lot of the women have a history of trauma, some have been trafficked, had PTSD."

Dr Moore sees some incredibly complex cases, and said that the cultural meaning of depression differs, so her work requires great sensitivity. "Lots of cultures don't recognise depression as a concept, patients present with physical complaints, when it's really about low mood which they can't voice." She comes across as passionate about the importance of supporting women throughout the perinatal period, and feels that lots of healthcare professionals still don't fully appreciate the significance of that time in women's lives, failing to see the risks of not adequately helping women. "It's also about the children, I can see so clearly and so quickly how the children are being affected. There is a sense of urgency, of wanting to treat people well so there is no long-term impact on the kids." Despite this, we talked about my perception that there does seem to be an increased awareness of PND. I said I felt like maybe more people are confronting their PND, but I wondered if talking about the effect on children could make people retreat and revert to keeping it hidden. Like Dr Belgrave, and the psychiatric nurses I met from the Bethlem MBU, she acknowledged that a key fear for a mother is having her child taken away. "It's proven in research, it's the deepest darkest fear. It is difficult to walk that line: talking about how it might impact on the children, without mothers becoming fearful that might mean social care being involved". But she explained that building a relationship with patients can ensure that women know that is not what is happening: that the aim is to support and protect the family. I'm curious about diagnosis, and the things which hamper it on both the patient and the professional's side – so we moved on to talking about the infamous Edinburgh Scale: the "quiz" which helps doctors and health visitors assess a new mother's mood. I mentioned that women (including myself) probably second guess what the professionals are getting at when they ask the questions, so presumably it's open to being hugely skewed? What did Dr Moore think of it?

"We don't use it in our service but it's a quick and easy tool in the community for a GP or Health Visitor. It provides a crude score but we would want to understand the symptoms and presentation in more depth."

She explained it's really a part of the assessment picture, not all of it: diagnosis cannot be just a numbers game – it is about evaluating the state of mind of the person sitting in front of you. With skill and experience a professional can see the whole picture – not just a snapshot of that moment when the woman answers the set questions. So many women I have spoken to admit to lying in their answers. And some of what is covered in the questions is part of the common experience of motherhood. Dr Moore suggests that unless there is a good relationship between the mum and the healthcare professional, there's a good chance women will not disclose the truth about their feelings, if they are negative: "If you're having dark, black thoughts – some women won't tick the answers, it's too frightening to admit them. You can't beat someone gently asking, really asking. A lot of women find it an immense relief [to admit their feelings]: it can be really powerful for them to let go." She commented that some women will just spontaneously tell you, but that for many it is harder, and perhaps they've never told anyone before. She reflected that if a woman is being asked questions about her mood at a busy baby clinic, perhaps with the door open and the next mum outside waiting, she's probably unlikely to confide in that situation.

"Often better quality referrals come from people who have an existing relationship: a GP the mum knows well, a family member who's brought them for help". This reminded me of an idea I had come across when working on older people's issues for a client. Among older people's support groups there is a concept people refer to – that of "noticers" or "befrienders" – the people who notice the isolated pensioner who perhaps hasn't turned up to the lunch club, or has clearly injured themselves in a fall but has no immediate family to look out for them and tell them to see a doctor. It struck me that new mums – new parents in fact – are perhaps in a similarly, if shorter-term, vulnerable position, and can benefit from "noticers" to alert professionals when help is required.

The Royal College of General Practitioners has produced an "Implementation Tool" on its website, to aid GPs in putting updated NICE Guidelines into practice. A section of this stood out (and I think all the women represented in this book would cheer if they read it):

"Recognise the exceptional opportunity of the 6-8 week maternal postnatal examination. This may be the only time you, as a GP, see a mother in the entire pregnancy and postnatal period. Consider asking about possible mental health illness BEFORE focusing on the physical tasks. Consider doing the mother's postnatal at a different time from the baby check. Disclosure is a 'red flag'. It's so difficult for a woman to raise this with a GP; if she says she has a problem, assume she does. Do not dismiss her."[2]

I discussed health visitors with Dr Moore, and she said, unsurprisingly, that it is very tough for them currently. There are not enough of them, and those who are there have enormous caseloads: "they're fire fighting really." In Tower Hamlets there is a proposal to make Health Visitors "perinatal champions" which sounds like a very positive step. We talked about how, for some women, even getting out of the house is such a challenge – as I well remember – and it is sad that

---

2 Practical Implications for primary care of the NICE guideline CG192 Antenatal and postnatal mental health - Dr Judy Shakespeare, www.rcgp.org.uk

the option of home visits just is not feasible in many cases. Dr Moore was very sympathetic to health visitors as a group, feeling they are overloaded. She also commented that some health visitors may feel unconfident in their skills around mental health support, even though they probably *are* skilled enough, but may be wary of asking the right questions.

Her team takes referrals from anyone – GP, midwife, health visitor, people known to community mental health teams, obstetricians. "What we want is to get women referred in pregnancy (women with a history). If the mother has had prior depression/prior PND or for example, bipolar, we want them to be referred in pregnancy. A lot are referred in very early pregnancy." I asked about recurrence – "You are more likely to relapse again in a second pregnancy but not all women do with good support and care around them. As a gold standard, if you've had significant PND that's required treatment, in a second pregnancy you should be seeing a perinatal psychiatrist – even if you're well." This was hard to hear, given my own experience second time around. It's probably the one line out of this entire book that I would love to see people remembering, quoting, and discussing.

During my pregnancy with Ted, I felt I had become depressed, and was feeling increasingly anxious. I felt I couldn't cope. I went to my midwives and GP for help, and was referred to the local hospital's perinatal psychiatric unit. I must say that subsequent experiences both there and at its sister mental health hospital have been wholly positive, so this episode is not illustrative of the level of support there. But it's what happened, and it sadly made all the difference. I had a relatively short appointment with the psychiatrist, in which I tried to explain what I was feeling, and why I was anxious about developing PND again. I wanted to know if I could start CBT as a preventative measure – and potentially start anti-depressants during the pregnancy, or immediately after the birth. Given what I know now, having spoken to Dr Moore, it's quite painful re-reading the letter the psychiatrist I saw sent to my GP, after he had seen me:

"Dear Dr ...

I assessed Ms Hargreave in the perinatal psychiatry clinic ... The reasons for referral were mild depressive symptoms in the context of a history of postnatal depression after giving birth to her first child in 2009.

Ms Hargreave had an episode of mild depression... following the death of her father. This resolved spontaneously. Ms Hargreave's first pregnancy was complicated with pre-eclampsia and ended with a complicated delivery and a 5 day stay on a busy postnatal ward. She became depressed within days of giving birth, presented to GP after 3 weeks, started taking sertraline 50mg OD after another week, and finally started improving after 4-5 weeks of treatment. The symptoms included persistent low mood, tearfulness, low energy, social withdrawal, pessimistic outlook and lack of motivation. There was no serious suicidal ideation or suicide attempt. There is no alcohol or drug abuse.

Ms Hargreave is presently well, with only minor worries and apprehension about the possibility that the postnatal depression might recur. There was a bout of mildly depressed mood several weeks ago, which passed spontaneously. Ms Hargreave presented as a smartly dressed lively pregnant woman, maintained good eye contact, spoke spontaneously with normal tempo and appropriate affective modulation. Her affect was fully reactive. Her sleep is disturbed by worries and physical discomfort of pregnancy. There was no sign of depressed mood or other psychopathology.

We have discussed the risk of recurrence of postnatal depression and possible preventative strategies. Given that there was only a single episode, which started in the context of severe complications and was not serious, preventive antidepressants are not indicated. Since there are no symptoms at present, cognitive behavioural therapy is not presently indicated. I only advise regular moderate physical exercise… and mindfulness training… that both reduce the likelihood of relapse. If mild to moderate symptoms of depression are present, please consider referring to Southwark Psychological Therapy service… there is presently no need for follow-up at the perinatal psychiatry clinic. If there are moderate to severe symptoms or other marked change in mental state, we would be happy to accept a re-referral…"

Re-reading this makes me feel pretty angry: not least because of the numerous inaccuracies in his narrative. It's possible I was just unfortunate that day, or that I misrepresented things too well. But given what Dr Moore later described to me as the women who she worries about – I think I was one of those women. Not suicidal, but certainly wearing "the mask". Dr Belgrave had explained to me that the concept of the mask or façade, especially with new mothers, is well known among mental health professionals.

Dr Moore talked about a patient who had a terrible experience of PND, but responded well to medication first time around. Second time around she decided to go straight back onto medication as soon as she had given birth. Others may opt to try without, but the perinatal team is there, monitoring and ready in case help is needed. I wondered if that was specific to Tower Hamlets. Dr Moore talked about the Royal College of Psychiatrists' (RCP) "perinatal community standards". There are 150 standards, which were developed by the perinatal quality network, which looks at all the services in the community. They cover who should be on the perinatal team, how to assess referrals. And there is a section about prior history. This is for people who *feel well during a current pregnancy but nevertheless have a relevant history.*

We returned to the subject of first-time mothers who are PND sufferers. "When it's a new onset... the woman has no experience of being a mum. She doesn't know what is normal." Her feeling is that the profession has done a lot of working on educating those on the front line about referrals, about recognising the signs. But she worries about other areas of the country, which perhaps don't have the same awareness. As well she might, given the map of perinatal care I was to discover later in my research.

"[in some areas]Women just get referred to generic psychiatrists who don't know about perinatal problems." The trouble with this is that perinatal mental illness is very particular, with a very particular associated risk: suicide.

I remembered one of the handouts Dr Belgrave gave me which touched on new mums who commit suicide. Dr Moore quoted a figure of around 80 women in a three year period who kill themselves.[3] "If you look at the women who kill themselves, it's very different demographically to people who normally self-harm. These women are in their 30s and 40s, from a higher class, they work, they are married, some will have a psychiatric history, but not all. The way these mothers kill themselves is also very different: much more violent, so hanging, stabbing – they're not superficial attempts. I don't think a lot of people get that. If I see someone in their 30s who's married, who's working, who's getting depressed: that's

---

3 Centre for Maternal and Child Enquiries (CMACE)

the woman I really worry about. To a GP they'll see middle class, eloquent, educated, someone hiding symptoms. To me that's the woman to watch."

What she said rang very true. Fortunately neither I, nor many of the case studies who share their stories here, reached the point where we felt suicidal. But the idea that many of us were adept at hiding symptoms was evident. After I met Dr Moore, I was so struck by this comment that I repeated it to some of the women who were giving me their stories. Whenever I described the "type" she had outlined, most of them said, "That's me." Personally, and it may seem a trivial point, but I would be willing to campaign to stop healthcare professionals asking "And how are you in yourself?" And that's not because I'm an English language pedant, although it does grate because it makes no sense, but because it doesn't really *ask* anything. And how easy is it to deflect a question that's not being asked properly? Too easy.

Dr Moore told me more about this type. "It's that thing of... 'oh, they're married, they've got support'. There's an over-reliance on that. It's the woman everyone else looks at and thinks they're coping. People don't really know about that specific profile." She mentioned a case, a woman she saw after her first baby, whom she asked to see very quickly having seen her case details. It was fortunate she did: she was already considering hanging herself, just a few weeks after the birth. In her opinion, this disastrous outcome was pre-empted by a good GP, who already had a strong relationship with the patient.

I thought out loud about a theme which seems to crop up with many PND stories: the feeling that "I don't want to be here". That's very different to suicidal intent, I assume? She said yes, it is. But though the suicidal mothers make up a relatively small number, they're not necessarily the ones who have psychosis. "With some women it can become a psychosis, but with some it's a rapid, severe depression. You can have suicidal intent and not be psychotic."

We also spoke about taking medication during pregnancy, another fascination of mine given my own regrets on not pursuing it as an option. It seems to be a controversial issue: some GPs won't even entertain it, and as my letter from the perinatal psychiatrist showed, specialists may concur, depending on the situation. That last point is the clincher, Dr Moore stressed. "You have to look at the individual case. You want a really thorough discussion with that woman and her partner, so that you feel it is an informed decision. Look at the risk, how severe [their previous PND was], has the mother been an inpatient, has she only ever been well on anti-depressants, and has she stopped medication? That's the guide as to how likely women are to stay well. What you don't want is someone to acutely stop medication without discussion." Having said that "We do use anti-depressants widely, we don't overuse them, we are cautious, but we are prescribing them routinely. There's growing evidence that they are moderately safe. In practice I have seen hundreds and hundreds of women take them and not seen effects on the baby." She says that the profession is aware there is a mildly increased risk of cardiac issues, but also says she has never seen this in seven years of perinatal specialism. There is also a very rare outcome called Persistent Pulmonary Hypertension (PPHT) in the newborn baby, about which there is conflicting data. Paramount, of course, is full disclosure. Patients are advised of the risks and given all the facts.

I mentioned that I'd had conversations with people who would caution against it because they feel there is enough evidence that it's damaging to the baby. "It does happen, but from my personal experience I've not seen it. What we do see more is some kind of withdrawal in the babies – they can be a bit jittery for the first few days. There is also conflicting data regarding autism caused by SSRI[4] use during pregnancy, but it's hard to prove whether it is linked to just having depression. My view is if you've got a mother who's had a significant long term history of depression, perhaps had hospital admissions, may have had self harm attempts in the past, has never come off anti-depressants: being realistic with these women, they would struggle to come off for that pregnancy, and doing so would increase the chances of them being profoundly depressed which brings its own risks." She did stress that obviously she would never pressurise a woman to go on anti-depressants, and would always support a woman in whatever choice she made. In fact she had patients on her books at the time who fell into all the categories – from a woman planning to recommence medication the minute she gave birth, to a woman who wanted to avoid it, but felt secure knowing the perinatal team were monitoring her.

I talked about a woman I'd met who developed depression during her first pregnancy: antenatal depression. I was interested in the perceived risks of embarking on anti depressants for the first time during pregnancy. Dr Moore said she would offer therapy in first instance - "CBT can be really helpful, really quickly" – but while some women manage to deliver without taking medication – some do have to. She said they don't have many patients on medication in pregnancy, but there are some cases where it is "the only treatment option. I've seen women deteriorate so quickly."

---

4 Selective Serotonin Reuptake Inhibitor, a type of anti-depressant

It is also a case of avoiding hospital admission if possible, and walking the line between pre-emptive action and heavy handedness.

Dr Moore stressed how important a supportive partner is. I remembered how much I needed Ben to give me license to take the medication. "Take the pills!" he urged me after the collapse which precipitated my starting Sertraline, one of his most memorable text messages to me in our entire relationship.

We returned to the subject of causes of PND: cultural, environmental, and circumstantial. From talking to Dr Belgrave and Dr Moore, I learnt that causes can be categorised by mental health professionals in three ways: biological, psychological, sociological. The biological link with PND is clear: some people have a genetic predisposition, with a strong family history of depression, or PND in particular. This is particularly the case if they have an existing bipolar condition or a relative who does. But also, crucially, so much is happening in a woman's body before, during and after giving birth. In my layman's view, "the hormones are all over the place", and Dr Moore agreed. "The dramatic hormonal shifts that occur immediately post birth, really fluctuating levels of hormones can trigger mood changes." I mentioned that for me it had felt like some feelings were extraneous, circumstantial, and some felt more like something taking over my body, a mood change I had no understanding of. I have likened it in the past to extremely severe pre-menstrual tension (PMT). She said it's often probably a combination (of the external and the internal). Are there psychological elements to do with personality, temperament, what our coping skills are like, and what has happened in the past? Was there a traumatic childhood?

The social elements are of equal importance. Often this is about what a mother's support network might look like. "For me, the biggest thing that's protective is social support, particularly in a second pregnancy". Where a woman is living, e.g. if she in a remote area, obviously her income and her standard of living, will all be factors.

I went back to the idea of the biological side of PND. I know that many women who have had it are keen to explore it, because they feel that it in some way vindicates them and backs up the sentiment that it is an illness, just like any physical ailment. In fact, Dr Moore says it is common for a patient to ask to have their thyroid checked, because they are so keen to prove they are not mentally unwell but instead suffering from something physical which is affecting their mood. Which in a way they are, just not in the way they think, or in a way which many find easy to talk about.

"There is a pronounced, marked change after birth (in a woman's body) which clearly affects mood. It's really terrifying for women, they literally think they are going insane. They've never experienced anything like that before, particularly puerperal psychosis."

I asked about men with PND, and, although the Tower Hamlets service is primarily for women, Dr Moore agreed it's definitely an issue, that men often experience depression as irritability "rather than a classic low mood" – so they might think they're just tired. She mentioned there are support groups, phone lines, and we had both seen some of the recent media coverage on the issue. I wondered if men find it harder to confront because they don't have the biological reason (excuse?) that women have. "Men have exactly the same stresses as women at that time" said Dr Moore – though we agreed that the physical changes are what separate men and women.

A few years back I had noticed PTSD being mentioned in the same breath as PND, and people starting to talk about the distinction between the two. I had talked to Dr Belgrave about it, and brought it up with Dr Moore too. Dr Moore explained that sometimes off-hand comments made by healthcare professionals around the time of the birth can haunt women, and affect them adversely. Dr Belgrave had met a new mum, whose baby a doctor had casually said was "lucky to be alive" – an off the cuff remark which caused a lot of anxiety afterwards. She felt this was reflective of a maternity culture in which the object is to "get the baby out", with often little thought for any resulting trauma.

I raised the "birth plan" concept with Dr Moore, who said wryly that it is her "pet hate." She can of course see the merits of it, but has clearly seen the problems it can cause if patients are not encouraged to view it as a flexible plan. "For some women [a birth plan] is not a good thing: they are fixated on what didn't happen, and can feel they have failed… some women are ok with it, they accept this is how it had to be". PTSD is one of her areas of expertise, and she says that there is definitely a growing awareness of it. In the past a lot of women were categorised as having PND, when in fact they probably had PTSD. Dr Moore believes that the experience on the post-natal ward doesn't help, and can mark the first stages of feeling traumatised.

Women are not necessarily getting "gentle, warm, supportive debriefing" which in an ideal world they would – instead they may be "belittled" or not heard. This means for some women things are left to fester. They may start rerunning the birth in their mind, having flashbacks and then having difficulty bonding with their baby. She explains that it takes a skilled professional to pick up on some of these PTSD symptoms, unless the mother readily gives up the information. And these are ideas and issues which can come to the fore again in a subsequent pregnancy.

We discussed the maternal choice on caesarean-section issues (given the NICE 2011 guidance on this). As it happened, when we met Dr Moore had just had a patient with a planned C-section for her second birth – because the first was "subjectively traumatic". I jumped on that phrase because it contradicted my long-held assumption that unless a birth is medically traumatic, there can be no link to PTSD. I remember discussing both my births with midwives at debriefs I had requested, and particularly with the first the midwife insisted it had not been in any way out of the ordinary. But what Dr Moore was saying was that even if it was not technically a difficult birth, she and her colleagues respect the woman's experience of it. "PTSD is about the perceived trauma – not what actually happened – it's how it felt. It might not be medically difficult in any way. It might be the way someone spoke to them." It may also be something key that happened in those early days. I can remember all too well each negative remark made to me on the post-natal ward after my first son's birth. And again, when my second was born, and I was desperate to leave the hospital (to avoid the trauma I felt first time around), but my blood pressure had yet to stabilise, the community midwife whose care I was under told me that if I forced the issue I may be referred to social services, i.e. I was not demonstrating a responsible attitude towards my new child by trying to discharge myself too soon. I remember crumpling when I heard those words. Fortunately another community midwife understood the precarious situation I was in emotionally, and colluded with a very understanding ward sister to arrange my swift release.

For the record, the NICE updated guidelines on perinatal mental health define traumatic births as "…preterm or full term, which are physically traumatic (for example, instrumental or assisted deliveries or emergency caesarean sections, severe perineal tears, postpartum haemorrhage) *and births that are experienced as traumatic, even when the delivery is obstetrically straightforward.*" (My italics).

I have never felt so alone as I did during the painful, interminable first week of my first son's life. I do wonder now about PTSD after my first, and possibly even my second birth. With my first labour debrief, I hoped this would lay to rest some ghosts, and perhaps it did. Second time around I was confused. What had happened to the wonderful second birth I'd been told so much about? The internet is rife with stories of women who had a terrible "medicalised" first birth, then took ownership of their bodies (or similar natural birth rhetoric) and managed a second birth which was very healing, much more positive, and exorcised the trauma of the first. If I sound flippant, I don't mean to be. I'm genuinely happy for people who this happened to, and some of their stories are shared in this book. I did dither a bit over how to handle my second pregnancy and birth, and in the end I decided once more to try for a home birth, and I chose another (different) team of community midwives to help me in this. They had specialisms in both home births and mental health issues, so seemed ideal. And, to be fair to them, they were great. But, I just don't think that for me it was the right choice. For whatever reason, my second birth, though considerably shorter than my first, was almost identical in how it felt: the same relatively manageable first half or so; the same almost tangible step when the contractions seemed to tip from difficult but bearable to completely intolerable. Second time around, I was labouring at home when the midwife thought she'd check my blood pressure. This was particularly important given my history of pre-eclampsia. Disaster: it was sky high. I had to be rushed by ambulance into hospital, and at this point my frail grip on managing the pain was broken. I can remember half the street coming out to have a nose whilst I hung off a railing in the ambulance, like a carcass hanging off a butcher's hook. With absolutely no irony, the paramedic urged me to sit down when the ambulance started moving, "for health and safety" reasons. I would have laughed if I had been able to. On arrival at hospital I demanded an epidural, which staff were reluctant to administer given that I was fully dilated, or very close to it. I insisted, and received it – it didn't work. I remember standing up to demonstrate that my legs were still working. Sadly, having had the epidural, I had all the down sides of it – i.e. being tethered to the bed and with monitors all over the place. But the real trauma for me came later, during a pushing stage which seemed to last forever and ended in another assisted delivery (ventouse this time). There was a stage when the midwives were effectively ushered to the side and the doctors took over, and not for the first time I found myself caught in the crossfire of their diametrically opposed views on how to proceed.

I was discussing this with a friend who was heavily pregnant with her third baby, and she mentioned a controversial video doing the rounds, of a woman giving birth in the US who was given an episiotomy without her consent. My friend described it as a horrific thing to watch, not least because of the bullying manner in which the doctor talks to his patient. This brought back a striking memory: a male registrar almost shouting at me to push. My recollection is that he was incredibly harsh, and certainly I can remember Ben stepping in at one point and saying something along the lines of "ok, ok! I think she gets it".

From what I've learnt in researching this book, it's quite possible I had PTSD after this birth too. Just as I find it harder to remember the details of PND second time around, the second birth for me is less defined in my memory. I was so happy when it was over, and I was so happy that it looked as though I would be out of hospital very soon – and that, this time around, Ben could stay with me. Even though he slept on an armchair by my side, the benefit of having him there is hard to quantify. I was high on adrenalin, the baby had latched on (a miracle, for me), and I held him on me all night, waiting to be able to text friends. But as the dawn came, I started to replay the birth and feel sick about it. I felt as though I had been cheated of the positive second birth I'd been hoping for. I told friends about this in a barrage of text messages, I had emotional incontinence and was fixated with the fact it had "gone wrong". When asked how, I couldn't explain – and this is where Dr Moore's explanation of the subjectivity of PTSD makes a lot of sense to me.

The way Dr Moore describes her unit is the definition of "joined up", the holy grail of healthcare we are all chasing, it feels, as patients. She is modest about this, and says it's actually quite simple: a key step being to ensure that everyone attends a team meeting once a week: health visitors, midwives, psychiatrists, psychologists, obstetricians. She calls them a "superteam". That one meeting saves everyone a lot of time, and a lot of chasing. Dr Moore's passion about getting it right, and avoiding the tragic outcomes of untreated severe PND, is palpable. She understands that flexibility is needed in how different women are treated, for instance, making it possible for a mum to be seen at home if getting out to an appointment was a challenge. Remembering the drama involved when I first went to a doctor's appointment with Joe on my own, I can see how welcome this option would be to many women. Rather than congratulating herself on her work, Dr Moore's attitude is more pragmatic. She points out that the NICE Guidelines say someone experiencing anxiety should have therapy within two weeks, and that often, in cases of new mothers committing suicide, there is evidence of a lack of communication between teams. She quoted the LSE report produced for the Maternal Mental Health Alliance (MMHA) campaign "Everyone's Business", from October 2014 about the cost to the NHS of maternal mental health issues. See Chapter 13 for more on what the MMHA and individual charities are doing on this issue.

The clinical psychologist

When I first became a mum, I longed for a group where I could go and talk honestly about the difficulties I was having, perhaps somewhere with professional help. So I was very interested when I noticed a psychologist advertising just such a group on local forums and Facebook. I went to meet her to find out more about her work. Dr Langhoff is a clinical psychologist who, like Dr Belgrave, works in both the NHS and private practice. In the latter case she is a perinatal specialist, so that was the work we talked most about – and that was what led her to try to set up a group for new mums, though interestingly she told me that she has had to put the group on hold for now, due to limited take-up. We talked about why that might be: I know I would have found such a group incredibly useful, but perhaps not all new mothers who are struggling feel that way. There are many reasons why they might not feel able or willing to attend. But, given that Dr Langhoff was offering the group for free, I was sad to hear she had not had more interest, particularly after I had talked to her at length about PND and realised how much she has to offer to people going through it.

Because Dr Langhoff's perinatal work is largely within the private sector, she says this accounts for about a third of her clients, simply because clearly many women cannot afford private therapy (although if they do have private medical insurance, her sessions are covered up to a point). As well as working with mothers, she does sessions for couples, both in the perinatal period and generally. That made sense to me, given how many of the women I have spoken to have talked about their relationships changing after having children.

In her work, she sees the whole gamut of perinatal presentations: antenatal anxiety and depression, previous birth trauma, mothers adapting to babies with disabilities (sometimes because of medical negligence during childbirth). She sees women with PND but also those who have adjustment difficulties to motherhood, which she thinks can last up to two years post-natally. She also sees mothers after their second or third baby, who have found that the new baby has tipped the balance. And she sees those who have suffered from psychosis, though this would generally be a bit further down the line, once they have had initial treatment on the NHS. This might not involve addressing the psychosis itself but the impact, the legacy of what it has meant for the mother and the family.

She works with a range of approaches: CBT for anxiety and depression, but also acceptance and commitment therapy, mindfulness, narrative therapy, systemic therapy. As part of her approach she allows couples to attend if appropriate, given how common it is for the relationship to be affected. "Every couple goes through an adjustment process when there is a baby. They are not really going out, sleep is disrupted, they may not be having sex any more. Something has changed. And then there may be different attitudes towards parenting." Sometimes it's helpful to have the partner there if the mother perceives them to have shown a lack of support, for example during the birth. A session with Dr Langhoff enables both to give their "side", so perhaps it transpires that the dad was occupied doing something he felt was of practical use (even if this was misguided.) Unlike my own therapy sessions, her clients usually bring their babies to therapy. She agreed that services which are not specialist perinatal therapies may not be flexible on this. When I started CBT, when my younger son was just nine weeks old, I was told from the start I could not bring him. Had I been still breast-feeding at this point it would have been very difficult. But my personal take on this was that it was helpful for me to have time away from the babies during therapy. Dr Langhoff had a different perspective on this.

"For me, some of the women have said it's reassuring bringing their baby. I can observe their relationship. Sometimes bonding might be affected, and we can talk about that and what things might be helpful for that. Some women find it difficult to talk in front of baby but usually it starts being ok. It adds a different dynamic, I will look at the baby too, I might hold them… it really works, and it enables women to come to therapy." She thinks it's unreasonable to expect a woman with a baby under six months to come alone to a session. She does give the option not to bring the baby, and it is sometimes discussed in sessions, but it has actually never happened, so clearly her approach works. She talked a lot about normalising, the importance of making this new life feel normal to the mother, and bringing the baby to sessions is part of this. I did query whether it might be difficult for women to share, for instance, invasive thoughts, in front of the baby. But her response was pragmatic:

"Baby is already witness to the distress and probably it's far worse than what will be coming up in my sessions, which are quite contained." Crucially, she is flexible: sessions can take place via Skype to enable them to go ahead if, for example, the baby is too sick to attend, or if the woman is at the point where just leaving the house is impossible. Incidentally, it's been incredibly comforting to note how often this problem comes up; even after years of reading and writing about PND, I had never realised how very much not alone I was in struggling so much to get out.

Back on her different approaches to therapy, she added that there is very good evidence to support CBT in the postnatal period, but also antenatally for anxiety and depression, and it is often the "first line of defence". This might be quite a brief piece of work. Often with PND issues, six to eight sessions is sufficient with a client, which is what is afforded on the NHS (although this does vary). She doesn't feel that there has to be a huge number of sessions. Despite the oft-quoted NICE Guidelines, she does find herself seeing women stuck on waiting lists for therapy on the NHS, who turn to the private sector if they are able to. Inevitably, by the time they come to the top of the waiting list they either don't want to leave the relationship they have formed with her, or they may no longer be in need of therapy.

Before commencing a course of therapy with a client, she has to work out what is important, and she will conduct an assessment to identify this. She has to disclose to the patient at this stage that the only circumstances in which patient/ therapist confidentiality can be broken is if she believes the woman is at risk of harming herself or others. In reality, this rarely happens. She is clear that there is a difference between "suicidal ideation", a phrase I had seen in letters to my GP from mental health professionals, and actual plans to commit suicide.

She sees a lot of women with birth trauma, which she says CBT is very useful for treating. These are women who may be reliving the birth. An acceptance and commitment therapy approach may work well here too, again bringing in a partner who can help talk through their perspective of the birth itself. The woman's memory will be sketchy, and of course is just one version of events. It's useful to hear the partner's version too. CBT, mindfulness and systemic therapy can also be useful in helping women adjust to motherhood. But in addition to CBT, her view is that the client needs to look at where her expectations have come from. Was she convinced there was only one way to 'do' motherhood? Breast-feeding exclusively, having the perfect birth, weaning with organic produce all lovingly home prepared… where have those ideas come from? She comments that these preconceptions add up to a feeling that "there is no way of getting it right, because there will always be someone in the media or in life with a different point of view. This is very important in terms of PND because it shapes our experience." Like other mothers, as well as health professionals I know, she finds it useful to invoke the "good enough mum" concept. This is a popular idea; in fact it now even has a musical named after it.[5] The

---

5 "The Good Enough Mums Club: It's ok to be a bit crap" – Giulia Rhodes, The Guardian, 30 August 2014.

mantra allows mothers to feel that they do not need to be perfect, they just need to be *enough*. I first heard it when Joe was just a few weeks old, from my community midwife. What would a good enough parent do? I told her about the "dare to be average" maxim I adopted after doing CBT, and she said they are basically the same idea. She uses this concept to help clients carry out small experiments, and to try doing things a bit differently in order to challenge less flexible thoughts about how parenting should be done. They will work on coping strategies: drawing on a woman's support network, but also helping her to expand it. That might be suggesting groups she thinks would be helpful for them to attend (which is why being a local mum herself is very helpful).

"Often the clients I see here are very career-focused generally, coming from a really structured, high powered work environment. How can you access local playgroups, how can you make mummy friends and not get drawn into the comparisons? Is it ok to be late for a group? These are very normal small scale discussions lots of mums have difficulties with – but the difficulties are heightened if you are depressed." I think her final point here is key. So much of what I felt was really more the sum of the parts, and the fact I was dealing with all of it in the context of depression (as well as external factors). Yet I remember how isolating it was when, seeking solidarity (and, if I'm honest, sympathy), I would put forward some of these feelings only to have some fellow mums dismiss them saying, "oh it's like that for all of us". Get over it, basically.

The talk of expectations inevitably made me wonder if she was alluding to the NCT. But she is diplomatic, saying it is more a feeling that comes from the media in general – the "Breast is best" rhetoric, for example, and the emphasis on the importance of routines. "The books saying you can get them into this routine if only you try hard enough. People read so much stuff and it really shapes some of the views. Some books more helpful than others, those that focus on the relationship and taking your time."

I was a routine mum first time round. I felt that Joe actually led us into the routine, and the books merely confirmed what he was telling us he needed. But I did become a bit of a slave to it. I always thought it saved me: it meant I got regular breaks because his naps were reliable, and he slept through the night from three to nine months solidly (stopping when his ear problems kicked in, recommencing after he had grommets fitted at 15 months). Now I wonder if in fact it caused me more stress. I think perhaps it was initially helpful, because I needed order, and needed to know what to do… but thinking back to my helplessness when he wouldn't nap as expected, or didn't sleep as long as the books predicted, I do wonder if it was a double-edged sword. Life with Ted was necessarily far freer, in part because I had a toddler to manage, but also because as a refluxy baby I had to be led by him and sleep was never a big priority of his.

The majority of Dr Langhoff's clients will have been on, or will still be taking, anti-depressants. She says of course some women decide not to, and that is fine, it has to be an individual's decision. She finds most GPs are aware of what is and isn't safe with breast-feeding. In common with the professionals I had already talked to, she is open to medication being used during pregnancy, particularly for anxiety issues. She also made a useful point: that for some women, particularly if for instance they are suicidal, medication is very helpful in getting them to a point where they can go to therapy. I thought that was helpful as women sometimes seem to see it as an either/or choice, rather than two options which may complement each other. I related the conversation I'd had with Dr Moore about the women to watch regarding suicide. Did the women she sees "mask"? "Not always, because I do have to address suicide directly at the assessment stage, so it comes up. Women often have the idea that their baby is going to be taken away. That really doesn't actually come up: my main worry at that stage is for the woman; establishing what the suicidal ideation is – whether there are any (suicidal) plans, what strategies we need to put in place. It doesn't always come up in the first session, sometimes it comes up once a woman has built more of a relationship. Part of it is women find it very scary to have those thoughts – but it doesn't always mean they are at risk of committing suicide. Lots of people have suicidal thoughts when they are feeling low. It is very frightening."

Sharing any part of the PND experience can be challenging, even just talking about experiencing low mood. I know many of the women I interviewed for this book admitted they had told few, if any, people about what they were going through. I asked about this and how, as a therapist, Dr Langhoff approaches it.

"There are women who can hide their feelings very well. It's very common to put on a brave face when you are out and not talk about those things. I think lots of women don't talk about it. Even when people know I'm a psychologist it rarely comes up, even though the incidence is high so I know there will be a number of women who are struggling. That's one of the big things in sessions, I try and normalise those feelings – it's not easy for any mother. But also when you are depressed it becomes even harder. How can you share this with people? Can you share it with your NCT friends?

Usually when women have the courage to share it they find others have similar feelings. It is a big step towards feeling better, once you are able to talk about it and get help, or get someone to listen."

She touched on tokophobia, which I had recently been reading about, and which Annie (Chapter 7) feels she suffered from. It's not something she has seen in private practice, though more commonly she might get people who are worried about the birth because of a previous bad experience, or because of family or cultural expectations. What she does depends on what the client wants: do they want to be able to have a different birth, or is it that they need to feel ok with the decision they have taken? The treatment is driven by this, not by the therapist's own agenda. She endorses hypnobirthing to help cope with birth trauma, and underwent it herself in her second pregnancy when she discovered very late on that her baby was breech.

She doesn't use the PHQ-9 or GAD-7 scale necessarily, but instead chooses to carry out a "mini review" at every session, to help clients evaluate their progress. She described a ruler concept, from solution-focused therapy, where the client is encouraged to rate how they feel at the start and then at the end of therapy: "sometimes people just don't feel confident, even when I can see they are much better. Part of my role is getting people to 'be their own therapist', and to be more able to recognise their achievements." She also explained the concept of therapists "cheering on change", which she does a lot of. "Getting people to notice things that are better can be really helpful."

Dr Langhoff works and lives in the same area of London, which inevitably means bumping into clients and ex clients while out and about, often with her own children. I've known therapists who find this awkward, but she is very relaxed about it. She says hello if someone comes up, they see each other's children. She sees it as a positive, saying it makes things more personal. She thinks it is helpful "to be normal, to say how's it going? just like any person, some people give you a hug", but acknowledges, "There are stances which are very different."

We returned to the subject of why the group she initiated had not really worked out. She says she tried, and she did it for a while, but there was just very little interest in it. She thinks there are various reasons, including finding a time to suit everyone. She also had to fit it in with her day job (the group was a free service). There are other groups in existence, including a local positive birth group, which has been successful. Perhaps there is a stigma in terms of owning some of the difficulties

I felt I had to ask about Dr Langhoff's personal experience, not least because she was sitting with her beautiful six month old baby girl, whose happy gurgling I can hear when I play back the interview. As with her position on bumping into clients, she is very open about her own experiences as a mother. She has had two children, and remembers that her first birth "wasn't great", and that breastfeeding first time around was very hard, to the point that she thought she might be on the brink of PND, but it did not develop.

In her second pregnancy she felt she catastrophised about feeling low in mood during the first trimester. She was working very hard at the time, had a toddler to handle, and was considering whether she needed anti-depressants. Her midwife told her to wait a month, which she remembers felt like a very long time. She was concerned about developing PND, because, as a therapist, she knew she was likely to, having had some low mood during the pregnancy. Fortunately, the low mood passed, possibly because she took action: "I threw things at it". She is very conscious as a therapist that there are things you have to do proactively, such as nurturing your relationship. "I know it's really important to be going out and doing things... we make sure we have date nights, and feel comfortable with getting a babysitter." The couple have no family nearby, so this was non-negotiable.

The GP and perinatal care commissioner

Dr Tara George has several hats: GP, teacher, and commissioner of perinatal mental health services for Derbyshire. Having heard so many disheartening stories of women who feel they were victims of the postcode lottery when it came to perinatal care, hearing about Dr George's work in Derbyshire was a very welcome change. Her role in commissioning came about when the local Clinical Commissioning Group (CCG) decided to ring-fence some funds for perinatal mental health, having identified inequality in the North of the county. The group wanted to offer a service to women in need, but they were smart: they knew they had to get an experienced GP (who happened to be a mother of two young children herself) to help ensure the services were appropriate. Would they be accessible, and would they be appropriate? Anecdotally, in her work as a GP, Dr George has a sense she sees more new mothers than perhaps an older male doctor would, and it definitely comes across that she is able to use her own experiences of motherhood to help put patients at ease when discussing what are often very difficult subjects. What she is part of in Derbyshire is, she believes, unique. They have set up a perinatal service which includes a dedicated perinatal psychiatrist and two Community Psychiatric Nurses (CPNs). Alongside this, they have formally contracted the services of the charity Family Action, whose role is low-level intervention. The two arms of the service seem to work very smoothly together. The services of Family Action are paid for out of the area's health budget, which seems to be a very enlightened approach to commissioning.

Dr George explained that Family Action provide help from the local Children's Centre in Chesterfield. They take both referrals and self-referrals, and, she feels, they fulfill an important role – often effectively the half way house between specialist perinatal help and no support at all. Some of their role is what she calls "befriending", akin to the noticing function I had been ruminating on after I talked to Dr Moore at Mile End Hospital. They are there to notice, for instance, that a mother may need specialist attention, and they can literally make the call to the nurse for her. The charity also focuses on confidence-building, and uses some low-level CBT techniques to help with this. That might involve setting a goal, and helping a mother achieve it – such as attending a local baby group. They may even accompany the mother to help her build her confidence.

As well as the work within Derbyshire perinatal mental health provision, Dr George's insights as a GP were intriguing. A very positive point she made was that post-natal depression is not a chronic condition. "Almost everyone will get better", and she stressed, just as Dr Moore had, that a huge part of PND is biological – and that biological cause does dissipate as time passes. "This will get better." Like Dr Moore, she was careful but honest about the risks of not treating PND. "Untreated mental health problems... can have a poor outcome for the baby." But, crucially, there are preventative steps which can be taken. Dr Beckie Lang, from Tommy's, the baby charity, had told me about the recommendations that midwives should ask mothers about their state of mind during pregnancy. Dr George agreed, and said that the midwives in her area had specific training on this point, and can signpost help depending on the answers they got, but that more generally there is a risk that this becomes a tickbox exercise. Something she is passionate about is normalising PND. That's not to say she doesn't take it very seriously, as her work exemplifies, but she is a proponent of the "you are not alone" line, and often takes pains to explain to patients coming to her with PND that they are among many parents she has seen with these problems. She commented that the majority of women coming to her with PND symptoms do genuinely believe they have in some way failed. Put that way, her argument for "normalising" those feelings is very compelling. Her approach as a doctor is "I'm the doctor: the response you are having is not uncommon. A lot of people feel like this and it is easy to think that because you feel awful, you must be deficient or not a good enough mother. [But] It's biology." She takes practical steps, pre-booking the next appointment for a fortnight's time, so that the mother has one less thing to do if she does need help… and, if the day comes and she feels fine, Dr George is still very happy to see her and confirm for herself that this is the case.

She is emphatic on the issue of medication. Not that she necessarily thinks everyone should take it, but that there is a dangerous level of misinformation in circulation about the safety of taking it either during pregnancy or while breast-feeding. "The vast majority of drugs for PND are totally safe in pregnancy and during breast-feeding." She worries that there are a worrying number of health professionals who simply are not up-to-date with the latest guidance on this. And so it's possible that mothers are being refused a treatment option because of their desire to breast-feed – when they may not have to make a choice. We discussed patients who may not want to take medication for other reasons – like Jill who was worried about getting too "used" to the effects. "[Patients] have several options. Do nothing. Take medication. Go for CBT or counselling. But at the point they see me, they may have struggled to even get out of the house to make their appointment. Their head may not yet be in the right place to benefit from therapy. Serotonin (increased by drugs known as SSRIs, e.g. Sertraline) boosts you, helping you to engage." Her words echoed what Dr Langhoff, the psychologist, had said to me – that sometimes people need the medication before they can reach a point where therapy is beneficial. As a GP, Dr George has to decide whether the patient will recover with "just" help from her GP and some additional help, or whether it is a situation where the perinatal team need to get involved. In accordance with the NICE Guidelines, her patients are seen relatively quickly by specialists when referred.

I questioned her a bit about suicidal thoughts. We so often hear about the GPs who get it wrong or don't ask the right questions, but clearly there are doctors out there like Dr George who don't take a standard form-filling approach. How does she see through the "mask of motherhood" I keep hearing about? "It's about asking the right questions. You have to be aware that people often hide things, especially people who have had babies. With the Edinburgh Scale… it's obvious what the 'right answers' are". As others have said, she understands that sometimes it's not about direct questions but about helping a mother to feel comfortable about revealing how she is really feeling. And of course, as a GP, she has a duty of care to the child – "Once you know, you can't un-know," she says of safeguarding concerns. But in fact, she has never had to involve social services – and she has treated many women with PND. "The majority have made a good recovery." When it comes to subsequent pregnancies, she takes a proactive approach: "The screening is automatically enhanced. There is a phone consultation with a CPN, and we really think about it: planning what the mother can do during the pregnancy. If she is struggling during the last trimester we might suggest she start Sertraline for the last eight weeks, and that might mean she is able to avoid being in crisis four weeks after the birth." Back to talking about medication, she remarks, "You take iron for anaemia." Meaning, why would you not treat depression, which after all has biological causes too? She agrees with Dr Moore that having a good relationship with your GP is very important to improving your chances of good mental health around motherhood.

When I re-read the MMHA Everyone's Business report, a line stood out to me, having spoken to Dr George: "Just 3% of Clinical Commissioning Groups (CCGs) in England have a strategy for commissioning perinatal mental health services and a large majority have no plans to develop one."[6] That makes what Dr George is doing in Derbyshire truly exemplary. I wanted to know a bit more about the Commissioner's viewpoint, so I spoke to Stacy Woodward, an NHS Commissioning Manager for mental health provision in Derbyshire.

Stacy informed me that there had been feedback following poor care in the north of the county. This, along with recommendations from the regional group on the

6 Everyone's Business report, October 2014

requirement for perinatal mental health services, and the variation in services across Derbyshire and the East Midlands, led to the Commissioners prioritising Community Perinatal Services. She added:

"As a general principle, we had already identified that we should not have special inpatient units in the area without having specialised Community Teams and in discussing if this is a priority, it was clear it was important to GPs, maternity units, social care and other providers."

Stacy explained that historically perinatal mental health services had not been commissioned in the north of Derbyshire. The south of Derbyshire, on the other hand, had a commissioned Community Perinatal Team. She started working with the Clinical Commissioning Group (CCG), back in 2013, and at the time, a project that had been established to develop perinatal services, co-led by Dr George, was in its early stages.

Stacy says she was conscious of the financial constraints within the NHS, and the project team had to think laterally about how they could address the gap they perceived in perinatal mental health care: on the mild to moderate end of the spectrum of PND. Stacy happened to live on the border with Nottinghamshire, and she knew about Family Action's work over the border there. She realised that Family Action could help fill the gap between low level to secondary services. She comments that not all patients requiring perinatal services may reach the threshold of secondary mental health services - and they are then left in the community and with the GP in primary care. She was impressed by Family Action's evidence-based approach, and following discussions across the North Derbyshire CCG, they agreed to commission Family Action. The vision was to implement a seamless service, from Family Action to secondary mental health services. Although it is still a relatively new service – and has not yet been formally evaluated – the anecdotal feedback is good. Stacy outlined to me the pathway that is now possible for a patient in the area: a mother might be referred for support with Family Action; but if she then requires a specialist intervention Family Action can refer her on to mental health services (the mental health team includes a psychiatrist, psychologist and community psychiatric nurses). Stacy emphasised that the gap Family Action fills is important on the way to recovery for people who have accessed the top tier of treatment -in-patients services.

Part of Stacy's challenge in setting up this innovative approach was pinpointing exactly where the patients were in the current mental health services. The commissioners ensured that Family Action was set up within the same building as the Community Perinatal Team (the Children's Centre). This helps to ensure that people do not slip through the cracks, for instance if they do not quite meet the threshold that is needed to be treated by the mental health team – then Family Action are right next door to help with some low-level support.

The project brings together all the professionals involved with perinatal mental health services – midwives, health visitors, social carers, Family Action, Sure Start and GPs. The project has also helped improve communications across all providers of care for these patients and this ensures that care is provided at the right place, at the right time, by the right person.

13

Perinatal mental health: the policy and the practice

Like any other area of health, perinatal mental health has a slew of stakeholders - from charities that provide services, to those which lobby for increased funding, and those who conduct research. I realised in talking to the mental health professionals that they all referenced the role that the not-for-profit sector plays in helping women like me and those described in this book. Having spoken to Dr George and Stacy Woodward, I also appreciated that the smart commissioning teams recognised the value of charities like Family Action. Some of these organisations are nationwide, some are local, but each has insight worth paying attention to.

Tommy's

My first conversation with someone in the sector was with Dr Beckie Lang, who is the Health and Research Manager at Tommy's, the baby charity. Tommy's funds research into problems in pregnancy and provides excellent general pregnancy information for all expectant mums. The charity was set up in 1992 by two obstetricians frustrated by the lack of answers around stillbirths, miscarriages and premature births.

Dr Lang works on a range of projects to support women to have a healthy pregnancy. One of these is mental health, a topic rarely covered well in pregnancy: many are more familiar with post-natal problems such as post-natal depression. Tommy's is keen to ensure that both mental and physical health in pregnancy are given equal focus and attention by women, health professionals, and society. Dr Lang explained that PND is really just one small part of the whole perinatal mental health picture. This is something I've slowly come to understand during the writing of this book: the spectrum includes not just PND, but anxiety, PTSD, antenatal depression, puerperal psychosis, tokophobia, obsessive-compulsive disorder plus psychotic disorders such as schizophrenia. To try to move antenatal mental health up the agenda, Tommy's joined the MMHA, an alliance I had already come across. She explained that the MMHA had been running for around three years, and in that time she has seen a change in the public perception of not just PND, but mental illness during pregnancy. Tommy's has been producing a lot of content around this, the aim being to help women take steps to pre-empt PND, by helping to address problems as they arise during pregnancy. Talking to Dr Lang I could see that this makes sense on many levels, the obvious being that prevention is better than cure. The impact on mothers, and their families, if they develop PND can be enormous. But there's also a pragmatic reason, a more mercurial one, which I've already touched on: it costs the country money. This is something that the MMHA realised early on, which is where their Everyone's Business campaign and report comes in.

Dr Lang told me that as well as their campaign, the MMHA has drawn up useful maps of perinatal care across the country. Having spoken to Dr Moore at Mile End Hospital, I was unsurprised to hear that Tower Hamlets is one of the areas of the country that stands out as having a high standard of perinatal care for women experiencing mental illness (marked green on the map). But the picture for the rest of us is bleak. Huge swathes of red across the country denote no specialist provision. [7]

Why is depression during pregnancy not known about? Dr Lang's suggestions were the sort which probably applied to the lack of awareness around PND not so very long ago: mothers feel fear, and may be afraid of their baby being taken away. Society expects this to be a blissful, glowing time, not one of dark thoughts. The mission for Tommy's on this subject is to raise awareness, and highlight the importance of good mental health during pregnancy and, importantly, ways of seeking help and support if your mental health is suffering during those nine months. She says, "It is OK to talk about it and we should be striving for no stigmatism around mental health. We don't judge women who have physical complications in pregnancy, so why should complications in mental health be any different?" Tommy's is working with the Royal College of Midwives (RCM) and the MMHA to create recommendations about the level of knowledge midwives should have on the topic of perinatal mental health, and they are committed to seeing the role of the Specialist Maternal Mental Health Midwife made available across the UK, but concede that until there is widespread take-up it is often down to the individual woman to tell her midwife what she is

---

7 everyonesbusiness.org.uk

feeling. This, Dr Lang explained, should "trigger a pathway" towards the appropriate help. It struck me as an effective pincer movement which Tommy's is sensibly campaigning for: encouraging women to take their concerns to their midwife or doctor, but at the same time urging the profession to spend more time checking on their patients' state of mind, and working with the MMHA to make the topic of perinatal mental health a priority with local commissioners.

Despite the bleak story told by the MMHA's Everyone's Business campaign, Dr Lang says the picture is changing, at least in terms of understanding around pregnancy and mental illness. She reports a perceptible change over the last two to three years. When I spoke to her the 2015 Election campaign was reaching a frenzy, and she mentioned that, for the first time, perinatal mental health issues had made it into each of the three main party election manifestoes. It was then borne out by the pre-election commitment of £75m over five years announced by Chancellor George Osborne in March 2015. On an anecdotal level, she has noticed that women are talking more about their experiences, which is something I've picked up on through social media. When I had my first son more than six years ago, it was definitely harder to find stories of people in similar positions. Now, you only need to search the hashtag "PND" on Twitter to see how many people out there are going through it, and crucially, talking about it. Dr Lang added that it's particularly powerful to see stories of women who have recovered. Her background is in nutrition, having trained as a public health nutritionist and then applied that expertise to public health campaigns. I had this in mind as I talked to her, and I was wondering what she felt about the feeding debate in the context of mental health. I asked her about it, explaining that I had noticed as I collated women's

PND stories how frequently feeding cropped up as, if not a trigger, then an exacerbator of depressive problems. She agreed, and said that despite her background in health and nutrition, and the fact that, for her, breast-feeding is "right up there" as a priority, that it must not be "at the expense of mum and baby." - an extremely reassuring, pragmatic response. Her thinking is that feeding, like many elements of pregnancy and childbirth needs support and encouragement. Not judgement.

We talked about the theme which has recurred throughout the writing of this book: that women who come to have their children later in life than our mothers did, have often been in work for many years beforehand, and may find parts of parenting, such as breast-feeding very difficult. The unpredictable elements to it can be hard for women used to being completely in control. The support still isn't there, according to Dr Lang, who wishes to see women getting the practical support they need to breast-feed into the labour and post-natal environments. She feels that many women are let down in this regard by a service that is under-resourced and over-stretched. I mentioned my realisation that it's not just breast-feeding issues which seem to compound depression, it's the baby's own feeding problems: for myself with my second son, and for others who have shared their stories in this book, issues such as reflux can have an enormous impact. Dr Lang agreed – although Tommy's focus is very much up to the birth, she has seen these problems in previous roles, and again refers to having appropriate support.

The idea of the birth plan, as I had discussed with Dr Moore, is not necessarily helpful. But what Dr Lang told me about sounded like common sense: she described the "wellbeing plan". This is endorsed by NICE, and the Royal College of General Practitioners (RCGP), and helps to encourage a discussion between women and their midwife or health visitor about what emotional support the woman may need. In drawing up the plan with her midwife, it affords each woman the opportunity to talk about her fears in a way which may feel less daunting than spontaneously mentioning her concerns in a routine appointment (how many of us have been on the verge of telling a midwife something during those precious appointments, only to back down or relegate it beneath physical concerns?). It's also an opportunity for midwives to identify those who many lack post-natal support, and help their patients start planning for after the birth. Wow, I thought. That sounds amazing. The trouble is it *is* amazing – and it's not part of the standard package yet. According to Dr Lang, there are areas of the UK that do use it, though the results on their success are not yet known. But informally, the feedback from Healthcare Professionals who have been using it has been very positive. A full evaluation is currently underway with City University, London.

Tommy's has launched some helpful advice on what is "normal" for emotional health during pregnancy, as well as some information on the most common mental health problems. Emotional health now features in its pregnancy calendar function, and they have also put together a series of short films looking at pregnancy mental health from different perspectives – women, partners, health professionals. These are all available on the Tommy's website, www.tommys.org/mentalhealth

MMHA

By now, I had heard about the MMHA's Everyone's Business campaign from a number of professionals and charities, and when it launched in July 2014 there was a huge buzz around it across social and conventional media. A report they commissioned found that the failure to properly address mental health problems both in pregnancy and in the first year following childbirth amounted to a staggering cost of £8.1 billion. The campaign press release explains that this figure relates to the "total economic and social long-term cost to society...for each one-year cohort of births in the UK". The report also found that almost three quarters of this cost (72%) related to adverse impact on the child, rather than the mother. Currently, according to the report headlines the average cost to society of one case of perinatal depression is around £74,000 (of which £23,000 relates to the mother and £51,000 relates to impact on the child.) The report argued that an NHS spend of £337 million a year would be enough to "bring the whole pathway of perinatal mental health care up to the level and standards recommended in national guidance. This is a case for investment that cannot be ignored."

And that case has not been ignored. In March 2015, the Chancellor of the Exchequer George Osborne revealed a large funding boost for perinatal mental health services: £75 million over five years. The MMHA welcomed this boost - while warning that future investment was required. They point to figures which suggest that more than one in ten women has mental illness during pregnancy or the first year after the birth, and that seven in ten hide or play down the severity of that illness.[8]

I spoke to Maria Bavetta, who is part of the Everyone's Business Campaign team. I knew how successful the MMHA had been in helping raise awareness, and had seen the

8 Boots Family Trust Alliance (2013) *Perinatal Mental Health Experiences of Women and Health Professionals an online survey of health professionals and mothers*

changes that were starting to come about, but I was curious to know how the sector had marshaled itself so effectively (when so many other groups don't). The alliance was founded by Dr Alain Gregoire, Consultant and Honorary Senior Lecturer in Perinatal Psychiatry (and now Chair of the Maternal Mental Health Alliance), from the Winchester Mother and Baby Unit. The alliance started with around six members – largely organisations who knew each other or worked together. But in the last three years it has grown exponentially: there are now nearly 80 members and counting. Members include specialist charities such as Action on Postpartum Psychosis and Maternal OCD, and large institutions such as all the Royal Colleges, NSPCC and Mind and even the state is represented in NHS England. What they have in common is a commitment to improving the wellbeing of mothers and babies. The value of that common aim has been recognized by funders: Comic Relief, and most recently Big Lottery have both granted significant funding to MMHA's work. When I spoke to Maria, they were half way through a three year campaign funded by Comic Relief, which focuses on improving specialist perinatal mental health services. "Our beneficiaries are mothers and their families, but our target audience is the decision makers", she said, recognizing that they cannot speak to every one, so they focus on the top tier of policymakers. Their work has focused on services mostly for women at the severe end of any perinatal mental health problem, although those on the mild-to-moderate end of the spectrum are by no means ignored, and as the alliance grows and takes on more campaigns, they are thinking of what they can do next. In fact, that seems very much their attitude: instead of resting on their laurels when the government funding boost came in, they are thinking "what can we do next, what bid do we have to write now?" in order to sustain their good work.

Maria talked about the Everyone's Business campaign's overall aim: to ensure all women receive the care they and their families need during pregnancy and the first year, as outlined in national guidelines. The ambition is to make this happen by 2020. The campaign has categorised their focus into three priorities they call their "Call to ACT", the acronym standing for Accountability – perinatal mental health care should be clearly set at a national level and complied with; Community – specialist perinatal mental health teams meeting national quality standards should be available for women in every area of the UK; and Training - training in perinatal mental health care should be delivered to all professionals involved in the care of women during pregnancy and the first year after birth. Scotland is currently the only UK nation which covers this within its healthcare training.

Maria says they regularly take calls from commissioners asking for help in promoting perinatal mental health in their area. The campaign team (Emily Slater, Campaign Manager and Maria Bavetta, Communications Officer) matches up these callers up with models of best practice, who pass on their learnings. The last year of the project will explore further ways to support perinatal mental health commissioners. As well as the specific goals they set themselves, MMHA also has a general aim around raising awareness and destigmatising perinatal mental illness.

Bluebell

I was gaining a clearer picture of what campaigners and researchers were doing on a national level. But I wanted to know too what a woman like myself might be able to access in a local context. As I'd seen, health provision varies wildly depending where you live. But springing up all over the UK are some incredibly forward-thinking PND charities. Dr Lang suggested I talk to the CEO of a Bristol-based charity called Bluebell Care. Ruth Jackson has a background in communications: she has headed up PR for some well known charities, but she set up Bluebell because she herself suffered from severe PND when her children (now aged 17 and 18) were born. She told me she had suffered from depression antenatally as well as post-natally. Although she had been living in London at the time, it had been impossible to access the appropriate care on the NHS, and she was fortunate to be able to pay for private help. In fact, she spent time at the Priory. Quite aside from her work on Bluebell, she has been informally supporting people in similar situations for the last 15 years. Before setting up Bluebell, which is based in Bristol where she now lives, Ruth carried out an extensive consultation with parents who had "lived experience", i.e. who had been through perinatal mental health issues. Her research covered a diverse catchment, including mothers, fathers, teenage parents, people from across the cultural spectrum, right across Bristol. The aim was to inform the service Bluebell would provide. She also put together a board, which included health professionals, and she says that from the start she never wanted Bluebell to be just about peer support. She was very emphatic that this is a delicate area, that any kind of peer support must be safe and supported, and that those delivering it need to be appropriately trained, with clinical supervision. She voiced her concerns that sometimes well-meaning people may seek to provide peer support before they themselves are well.

This was a perspective I hadn't considered before. It pulled me up short. Off and on, over the past six plus years, I have considered whether I should do anything more concerted than the occasional 'buddying' role I have played. And I do know people – like Sarah – who are doing this, but with the appropriate support. Now I realised that some of my vague ideas from the past – about setting up a forum, for example, to help depressed mums – were perhaps a little misguided, Ruth's point being that sometimes "peer supporters might not be fully prepared for the emotional impact supporting others can have on their own wellbeing and therefore need to be significantly recovered, ready, supported and prepared to take this on." So the Bluebell ethos is that everybody is properly trained.

They have two main services, and have fundraised to enable their delivery. They work largely with paid professionals, and only a handful of volunteers. They operate a therapeutic group programme: "mums comfort zone", a 12 week course run out of Children's Centres all year round. This is aimed at mothers who are struggling, or have already been diagnosed, with either ante- or post-natal depression. Often they are referred by their Health Visitors or GPs. The groups are led by an Occupational Therapist (OT), who did have PND. Another part of Bluebell's ethos is to stick to best practice in administering groups, so there is always a co-facilitator. These women are people who have also experienced perinatal mental illness, and work alongside the OT in the group. Participants also receive a toolkit, and the course itself is very structured. There is more of an emphasis on anxiety, because, Ruth's experience, like that of Dr Belgrave, is that more women present with anxiety than depression perinatally. The women are taught very simple strategies and coping techniques: relaxation, diaphragmatic breathing. A varied mix of activities, including music and art sessions, even some pampering, ensures that everyone is kept engaged.

Separately, Bluebell runs a buddy service. Each of the three co-facilitators has her own mobile and covers a different area of the city. They offer one-to-one home visiting, both to those attending group sessions, and those who do not feel they can. The buddies are peers, but they have specific listening skills, and have received training on safeguarding. They also crucially receive clinical supervision with a psychologist regularly, where they are able to reflect on the mothers they are working with, share any concerns and anxieties and receive feedback to support their own well being. They are not volunteers; these are paid roles. They may visit a woman six to eight times at home, and in between they will text or call them to check in.

As I had done with everyone working in perinatal mental health, I asked about the middle class, professional, suicidal mother Dr Moore had described to me. Ruth said that what they are seeing are more and more women who work in a particular field. These are women who have never told anyone they are suffering from mental illness. Despite our increased awareness and understanding of post-natal depression, there is a constituency of women accessing Bluebell's services who feel held back by the stigma, and are unable to tell people within their own profession, medicine.

Bluebell's services do not exclude men. They have a peer support group and one to one 'Buddy' support for men delivered by a trained peer support worker, who is also a dad with lived experience. Focus groups told them this was the help fathers were most keen to receive. Often it is just about reassuring dads that their partners will recover, and one day the woman they knew will return. There is, just like elsewhere in the country, a growing appreciation that partners' themselves may be vulnerable to depression.

So Bluebell is about far more than just some mentoring. It is squarely founded on evidence. And like any organisation which operates on evidence-based principles, it is subjected to evaluation to check on its results.

Family Action

Dr George had introduced me to Family Action, the charity she works with in Derbyshire. I later spoke to Sam Wilkinson, Perinatal Co-ordinator there, for her perspective on working with women with PND. I had a host of questions for her. I had been thinking a lot about how PND affects the whole family, not just the mother. Dr Langhoff had already told me that she sometimes treats couples together. Did this holistic approach make sense in a setting like Family Action? Sam said she does have contact with family members, in fact it is her preference as it allows her to work with the family as a unit. She carries out home visits which often means the dad may be at work when she calls, but when she has had the opportunity to meet them it has been a positive encounter. "They seem to really appreciate me engaging them in conversation and asking about their experience and I have found that they are then more supportive of the mothers embracing our service."

When we were nearing the end of our week of hell in hospital after our first son was born, Ben was touched when a kindly paediatrician showed concern for him and told him to make sure he got some rest. I remember being really irritated by that, but now, six and a half years on, I can see that this was probably the only time anyone (other than perhaps our family) showed concern for him, and the fact is he was exhausted just like I was. He was trying to keep the show on the road. And when we were told we could go home, he cried.

Interestingly, Sam says she also meets women's mothers, which is also positive, and she has found that they are often good at encouraging their daughters to take the help that is available. This whole family approach sounds crucial, particularly in cases like the disabled mother of three, whose 11 year old provides a lot of the day-to-day practical care. Family Action supports that family, and is helping the 11 year old as part of that. This means, for instance, a young volunteer taking the 11 year old out while Sam is helping the mother.

The women Sam sees generally fall into the "mild to moderate" category of PND. She works with GPs as necessary – sometimes taking referrals from them – and often updating them. Health visitors, midwives and children's centre workers are also able to refer to Family Action. "I also work closely with the psychiatric perinatal team which addresses the more severe cases of perinatal mental health. I feel this has been a necessary and successful partnership and I have delivered some groupwork with one of the psychiatric nurses which has supported mums from each of our caseloads."

Of all the things she does in her role, she suggests that the most helpful is "active listening… Often women don't necessarily want someone to 'fix' things or give them solutions but to have the opportunity to unpick and process things for themselves, so a safe and facilitative environment can be so powerful."

There are of course practical things the charity does too. And one of these, I was delighted to hear given my earlier thoughts on noticers, was volunteers who act as befrienders to ensure women are not isolated. So that might mean going with mums to baby groups or on general outings, which, as many of us know, can be so overwhelming to do on our own.

"The smallest of things can make the biggest difference… having someone to offload to, someone who can relate to parenting experiences, someone to hold the baby so mum can drink a cup of tea in peace, someone to pick up a family and take them to group and bring them home afterwards just reduces the stress and anxiety of getting out."

Sam says her service users "seem to cover the whole spectrum in terms of class, age, education…" She has mums who are very young but also older mums, professional career women and financially deprived women. "Perinatal depression does not discriminate in who it affects. A common denominator between every referred mum, however, is a degree of social isolation."

I asked Sam about antenatal referrals, and she says these are coming through now, and it's something she wants to encourage to happen earlier. "Many women who are referred after the birth acknowledge that they actually started to struggle during the pregnancy."

What must feel particularly gratifying to Sam, as well as to Dr George and the Clinical Commissioning Group who contracted Family Action, is that she reported women saying they felt the service "was the missing link in terms of getting the support they needed. Whilst medication is helpful, it isn't enough and a specialist service like ours really is needed to provide the emotional support women need during this vulnerable stage in their lives."

14

The mask of motherhood – why we lie

Isabel's story

Isabel has three children, and is one of many women I've spoken to who never told anyone (other than her partner) that she had PND. I asked her about the Health Visitor – had she checked the Edinburgh Scale questions with her? "Yes," she said. "I lied." On reflection, she feels she had significant PND with her first, and to a lesser degree with her second, but didn't have it with her third.

When she was pregnant with her first, she was living in a very isolated rural setting. She was new to the area and did not have local friends until later when she did her NCT classes and made a close circle of friends in the area that way, and says they were "each other's saviours". She remembers feeling mostly happy, but definitely lonely, and walking the dog a lot. She loves living in the country but says "small children and a very rural setting don't mix", especially when it's a bleak winter. She got to know her neighbour in the end, once her daughter was six months old.

The other thing she remembers making her feel low in the first pregnancy was that she suddenly developed acne, which she had forgotten all about until seeing some old pictures recently. She hated it, and felt shocked – she had expected to be glowing throughout, but in fact she felt nauseous throughout the pregnancy, and hated the change in her body shape. "It's like someone else's body... you lose all dignity, with the midwives prodding at you."

She opted for midwife-led care, which she was unable to repeat with her second and third children as she had a condition in her second pregnancy which necessitated consultant-led care. She was clear with her first birth that she did not want interventions, or doctors in the room. Her husband was nervous, but understood that the main thing was to support her. Her baby in the end was two weeks early, which she found quite shocking. It meant she missed her final NCT classes (including the one which covered breast-feeding – this happened to me too). She had a long labour, and was turned away from the birthing centre twice, and told to go home a third time but refused. She remembers the midwife being cross that she refused the gas and air (and pethidine), and telling her "we're running out of options". This was followed by a very long pushing stage – two hours – but quite a straightforward delivery. She was determined to avoid being catheterised, so went to the toilet frequently. She describes sitting on the toilet and thinking to herself, "this is the most horrific thing I've ever experienced." The contractions were intense, and she says "pure agony... I felt inhuman." Her mother had always painted a picture of both a blissful pregnancy and a wonderful birth, but this was not what Isabel experienced. That phrase, "the most horrific thing..." kept going round in her head throughout the rest of her labour. After the delivery, she delivered the placenta which she found to be the worst part in each of her three births. I remember feeling shocked by the pain of that too, after Ted's birth – there is a feeling of "will it never end?" She concludes that the first birth was "technically textbook... but so shocking for me. I felt like I'd been attacked." Which brought to mind what I had discussed with Dr Moore about subjectively traumatic births. Isabel's husband was able to stay overnight with her at the birthing centre. But feeding was difficult: the baby was small, and her mouth was tiny. She remembers "the midwife just grabbing my boob and the baby's head... there was no dignity here". Though she breast-fed each baby, she says she "never just took to it. It was painful, I didn't enjoy it." Again, her mum had given her the impression it was easy and enjoyable.

Unfortunately for Isabel, a family wedding when her baby was very young put a lot of additional pressure on the couple. Not only were they visited immediately after the birth, but in the weeks that followed there were a lot of extended family visits. She remembers that first visit in the birth centre, with her tummy still "massive", feeling "disgusting" and her in-laws cooing over the baby and all but ignoring her. Because her daughter was born early, it took a while for her NCT friends to catch up, so at first she was alone. She remembers that they did manage to get out, but it would take forever to get ready, and she was still in a lot of pain in those early days. There was an initial feeling of euphoria and adrenalin, but it wore off. She did feel very close to her husband, he was very supportive and did a lot to help out. Miraculously though the baby started sleeping through at six weeks. Despite this, the whole experience was still very tiring.

In the early days, before the baby slept through, her husband realised she wasn't coping on the lack of sleep, and would take the baby into the sitting room, and sleep on the sofa with her in her crib next to him. He would bring her in for her feeds, or sometimes she would express so he could bottle-feed at night. "Sometimes now I cuddle her, and remember the mornings when he would be going to work, I dreaded him opening the door and saying, 'Here she is!'" Her husband works shifts, and at six weeks he started doing nights, which is why it really was a miracle that the baby started to sleep through at that time. Despite this, she was a baby who "cried all the time" during the day, and it felt as though she was the only one among the NCT group who did. This, along with pressure from in-laws to visit whenever they felt like it, seems to have triggered the depression. But despite this she was adamant she would not talk to anyone, not even her GP. She felt her husband didn't want to approach it directly, other than a couple of tentative attempts. "I didn't want to accept help," she says, wondering whether this was because she herself is in the medical profession. Her GP was an unsympathetic character anyway, so she was unlikely to go to him for help. She can remember a friend confiding that she couldn't stop crying and felt like she was under a big black cloud. Instead of opening up about sharing those feelings, she tried to help her friend. She says she tends to prefer being in the supportive role to opening up. She also feels she was in denial: "I didn't think I had it", yet admits she had thoughts which scared her, like pushing the baby down the steps in her pushchair. She felt trapped in a house which was remote. She did finally admit to herself that she wasn't feeling "normal". "I wanted to be away from her all the time. [My husband] was terrified of leaving me." She resisted seeing a counsellor, having had a negative experience with one as a teenager. She also said there was no way she would tell her own mother how she was feeling.

It seems in retrospect that there were several key events which helped Isabel to recover. When her daughter was around six months old the family moved house, to a small village. Although it wasn't the main reason for choosing that village, one of her NCT friends lived there. She was not now going for days without talking to anyone. At nine months, the couple went away for a short break, leaving the baby with family. She felt judged by some of her peers for doing this, but she felt desperate and very much in need of it. She loved it, and says she didn't want to come back, although she did miss her little girl. But she felt it was important for the couple to get away, and they had a good break. Then when her daughter was 14 months old she went back to work, in a new role. She loved her new job. She said it was exciting and she felt so happy – and found she didn't miss her daughter at nursery, which most of her peers said they did.

When her daughter was around a year old she felt a sudden urge to have another child, and has had the same urge at the same time after each baby. She had one miscarriage, but conceived again straightaway. Despite being very new in her job, she was delighted. She was concerned about being depressed again, but generally she felt well. She had been dreading her second birth but was amazed to find that, though it was painful, it was less painful this time: "It was a breeze compared to the first time." Her second baby was very placid and did not cry much, and she enjoyed the early days. "I was tired, but I knew what to expect... I was totally unprepared first time around. I wish there was a book that told you about everything." She feels that some of the hard parts are not covered in classes or books, such as the after-pains she felt with increasing intensity after each birth. After her second baby, she was on a massive high – until the baby developed meningitis at five days old. They were in hospital for a week: "The worst week of my life". She had sensed something was wrong, the baby's cry hadn't sounded right and her temperature was high. Thankfully, she made a good recovery. For the first time, she voiced her concerns about depression out loud, saying to one of the nurses, "I'm terrified I'm getting PND again". As it happened, she felt ok for the first six months, when she felt she did have a dip, though not to the extent that she had it the first time. She wonders if this is because the second one was an easier baby, or because this time she had more of a support network in place. She says that dog-walking was something she found good for the soul; she did it twice a day and it helped to clear her head. Other than that, she thinks that really just time passing helped her recover.

I always credited my first recovery to the combination of anti-depressants, counselling and the support of friends and family. I also think taking on freelance work when Joe was a year old helped give me some of my life back. With Ted it's perhaps less clear-cut. I did return to work – to the job I had last done when pregnant with Joe – when Ted was about one. Shortly after that, we enrolled a sleep consultant to help us with his diabolical sleep. When I say he was a bad sleeper, I mean he was waking every 40 minutes. And we had tried everything. People sometimes said, oh why don't you co-sleep? We had been co-sleeping on and off since day one. At its worst, he was still waking every 40 minutes in bed with me. That's when we knew we needed help. We took a very very gentle (no cry) approach prescribed by the consultant, and it worked. It wasn't a miracle cure. He still took another year to sleep reliably but I would say it was a 50% improvement on the sleep we had been getting: just what I needed now I was back at work. Even though I only stayed in the job a year, before opting to go freelance for a better home-work balance, that year was definitely instrumental in helping my recovery. I probably thought I *was* better when I started back, but looking back, I was not. I think it would have been hard to be better on the little sleep I was getting, and given my pre-disposition.

15

The external factors we can't control

Lily's story

Lily has a son, who is now nine. She went into motherhood thinking that she would feel like part of a family unit, and that she and her husband would enjoy the experience together. She thought, "It might be fun… and certainly not destroying…" And she also felt that she would enjoy having a little person in her life. Of those thoughts, the last one came true, but the others did not. "I felt constantly scrutinised for 'only having one', so I didn't feel like a proper family." Lily had suffered from hyperemesis so severely she felt sure from the very outset that this would be her only child.

She comments that her husband's response to having a child felt very different to hers; she felt he was enjoying it far more than she was: "He seemed thrilled, delighted, proud of himself and our son and I didn't feel the same at all." She admits to feeling very isolated. But she is pragmatic, and she forced herself out to find the "mummy friends" we all hear we are meant to make. This, she feels, was helpful to some extent, but she did feel something of the odd one out. The mums she befriended were affluent, with a lot of financial and family support – Lily had neither. She uses the word "destroyed" more than once to describe how she felt with a newborn, saying this really kicked in at about three weeks. She had an undiagnosed dislocation at the base of her spine from the birth, which was not picked up until six months later when she broke her spine in an accident – two days after going back to work. She retains some positive memories despite these setbacks: "I did like having the little person in my life, and he was super smiley and often a great comfort in my daily misery and feeling of failure."

In addition to the physical setbacks Lily faced, she moved house when her son was just three weeks old. Her sister moved abroad. She was the first of her group of friends to have a baby. And the woman she called her "borrowed mum" died just before she got pregnant with her son. She was "drowning in grief". After moving house, she left behind her midwife, who she describes as "still one of the most important people I have had in my life. She was totally fantastic. She referred me to CRUSE bereavement counselling when I was around five months pregnant, and suggested she thought I had antenatal depression." Lily found this helpful but she had a big fear of PND, and knew that antenatal depression was a likely antecedent of it. So she did not want to confront the possibility that she was depressed – "I went into my shell quite a lot."

All of this followed a pregnancy which was highly fraught. She spent five months in total in hospital, in an assortment of wards, and hated it. She was sick every single day, sometimes up to 40 times a day. "I often felt people around me thought I just couldn't take it and ought to pull myself together. I lost my income (self-employed) and I felt miserable and isolated and teary a lot."

In contrast, and mercifully, the birth itself was good. She laboured mostly at home, then when the baby got stuck was transferred to hospital where he was eventually delivered in theatre – but with the midwife present.

Three weeks later and having moved to a new town, away from the brilliant midwife, Lily was seen by a health visitor at her new home. Lily remembers "She said 'I see you have a nice home – you're not really one of my priorities.' I cried a lot after she left."

By this point her partner, who had loved his two weeks of paternity leave, was back at work. She found the days exhausting: "frightening, isolating, a blur of sleep deprivation and physical pain."

I asked her to describe how PND felt – she replied "like I wasn't coping, and I should be. Like I didn't love my child (enough)." She did see her GP, who actually (unusually, given most case studies described here) pushed a diagnosis on her, and suggested she was in denial. She later read her medical notes through and found that very phrase "patient denies being depressed" was written down. She remembers with some amusement his admonition to her to get some more sleep. She had gone in on that occasion for mastitis, and says that in fact she did suspect depression herself, but that the GP did not agree. She's still unsure whether there was ever a formal diagnosis, but she did go home and regularly completed the Edinburgh Scale with her husband.

The things which Lily feels went well are perhaps the things that saved her – managing to get out, during a long hot summer: long seaside walks which she feels helped her mobility and physical recovery. She was very organised, and managed a routine, though not in the strict sense of that word. Her husband was a commuter and she would stay out late with the baby until he was home, and she managed to get him to sleep on the go which helped a lot in giving her a sense of freedom. In retrospect, she says very honestly that she feels her son saved her life. She thought of leaving when he was tiny and she was feeling overwhelmed: but the fact he was dependent on her for feeding stopped her.

The depression lingered. At 18 months she still felt depressed, partly due to an accumulation of fatigue. And even though her son is now nine, and in many ways she has moved on, she says, "I still feel a bit of a 'fraud' as a parent sometimes and I do feel scarred by the pregnancy and PND. I could never face it again and so didn't feel I could have another child. This was a factor in my separation seven years after our son was born (as were other things like commuting and personality) but it is a chunk of guilt I carry."

She is clear in her advice to others: work out a plan for practical help that you want, and that will really make a difference to you.

16

Away from Home

Alice's story

Alice is French Canadian, and moved over here when she was five months pregnant with her first son. Despite several extended visits to her partner over here, she had never lived here full-time (nor with her partner), so she dealt with a lot of change in what was already a period of considerable transition. In her home town the maternity provision is very poor, so her perception of the NHS is very positive. She enthuses about the access to GPs, midwives, local hospital and the liaison between all of them. On arriving in the UK, she settled in and signed up for NCT classes as a way of making new friends, although as English is not her first language she was struggling constantly with a language barrier. Her NCT group were nice, and she made good friends with them. She remembers her birth being "ok" – although on closer questioning it turns out she reached the pushing stage while still only in the waiting room at the hospital. She did manage to secure a private room on the ward, but nevertheless was plunged straight into "a breast-feeding nightmare". Like me, she was encouraged to use donor breastmilk. She struggled on with breast-feeding for five months. She describes her son crying and clearly very hungry as a newborn, although she does remember the midwives she had during that first month as being very attentive, a good support. She liked the breast-feeding cafes which were on offer locally (as I write these are now under threat), and said they helped to "break the isolation". She sought specialist help with the feeding, and even took pills to increase milk production, but the baby developed jaundice. She describes herself as being "stubborn" in her attitude to breast-feeding: she was determined to do it, and in fact it was her midwife who told her to be realistic, along with her mother, both of whom advised her to supplement with formula, which she finally did at five months. She says she felt guilty giving him a bottle in public.

Another unexpected outcome was the physical pain after the birth. She had assumed that would all dissipate after labour had finished. But the bleeding, the recovery, crying as she went to the toilet, she hadn't expected. The lack of sleep was a shock too. "With breast-feeding… I was crying all the time". Luckily her son was a good sleeper from about six months on. Her partner was working as a teaching assistant at the time so was able to be home after four o'clock most days which was a huge support: "He was really present". They took decisions communally, which in some ways she struggled with – the differing values held by each. The couple had gone from a long-distance, long-term relationship to living together in the same house and same country with a small baby in a short space of time.

Despite all these factors, she feels the stress levels she felt were relatively "normal" after her first son. It was after her second that she became actually depressed. He was born two years and two months after her first son. The birth itself was fine, again. But she felt she could not cope well.

"With the first one it's all new...with the second there is not the same excitement. I was tired, and [after he was born] impatient, would scream at my older son." Having a background in education, at the more progressive end of the spectrum, she had assumed she would be a great mother, and certainly not one who lost her temper. There was a feeling she was causing more damage than good. She doesn't feel she had the instinct to want to die, because she felt very strongly that her children needed her. But she looked at their relationship with their dad and felt it was stronger than the one they had with her. Although she did not feel suicidal, she did have thoughts of hurting herself, and felt uncertain if, for instance, she was near a knife in the kitchen. She stresses that for her, the problem was not with the baby. It was with herself. She describes what adds up to a loss of identity. Perhaps in part because she was living in a new country, but also the demands of a toddler and a new baby, made it hard for her to know who she was any more. She did visit her GP, who suggested anti-depressants, which she was not keen on. She opted instead for six sessions of "talking therapy". She wasn't very sure of her therapist, and feels six sessions are inadequate time to form a good relationship. It helped a bit, but she found the therapist "didactic... I found it hard to open up." She then explained to me that, unbeknownst to almost everyone other than her partner, she suffered from an eating disorder from when she was 11. At 14, she sought the help of a therapist, who sadly she found very invasive in his methods. This bad experience left her determined to "do it on my own". She left home at 16 and became very secretive. As a mum to two children, she found herself missing her freedom. This partly manifested in a desire to get out of the house and do something away from the children. Combined with feeling negative about her body (she wanted to lose three stone) she needed something new, and she found it in capoeira. She describes her involvement in this as "a godsend". She started it only a few months after her second son was born, and now practices it several nights a week. Despite this need to get out and do something, she is clear that being a full time mum is something she values highly. She never shared the sentiment of "missing using my brain" which new mothers discuss. She emphasises that as a parent you are using your brain. Or you should be.

Starting capoeira gave Alice "confidence. A connection with myself." She made friends, most of whom were childless, she felt she gained the best shape of her life, and she gained a new social circle. Her therapist, concerned about what was driving her, admonished her not to cheat, which, understandably, she found irritating (and possibly inappropriate on the part of the therapist). Her partner was very supportive of her taking on this new interest, as he could see it helped. She was able to find her own friends – not people connected with him, or her role as a mother. Having two young children meant she had got used to being tired, so energy levels weren't a problem. On the mental side, she has recently completed a course with the Kids Company, and is hoping to do one-to-one support in schools on the back of it. The course helped her too. But it has also made her reflect, and she worries about having damaged her children with the times she has lost patience in the past. "I can never erase it and now they will remember…"

Her description of the impact a new interest had on her depression made me think about how taking up Pilates when Ted was about a year old had really helped me. It gave me a space to do something that was actually fairly achievable, in that all the movements are small and nobody is urging you to blast the fat or run faster. But it was also practical: I suffered from diastasis recti (separated stomach muscles) after Ted was born and started Pilates in a desperate attempt to address it. It had become one of many obsessions, something I had to fix. Perhaps it wasn't the quick fix I wanted but it certainly worked, and in more ways than I had expected.

Looking back, she's not sure why she refused medication, but says in her home country medication is handed out to children with Attention Deficit Hyperactivity Disorder (ADHD) (in the schools she worked in) "like candy". Perhaps there was a lingering (negative) association for her. She was open about the therapy, but it's sad to hear that after her six sessions were up and she revisited her GP, he said – it wasn't a question – "are you better now". She said yes, and says there was nothing else on offer. She wasn't aware of other organisations or charities which might help. She points out that there is plenty of help in her area for breast-feeding – but not for mums with PND.

17

Pre-conceptions: when
mental health problems
strike before conception

Joanne's story

When I was planning this book, I was approached by
someone who had experienced great difficulty in
conceiving, until she finally did so after seven years of trying,
on her second round of IVF. She told me that while she had been
fortunate not to suffer from PND after the birth of her first child,
she had certainly experienced some form of depression and
great stress during her attempts to conceive. I was interested by
this, because whether or not it is unique to her, her difficulties
in having a child seem to have produced a very positive frame
of mind when it came to actually being a mother - in contrast
to my own experience, and that of so many described here. I
am sometimes wary of talking about PND with people who I
know have struggled to conceive: I fear they will perceive it as
somehow ungrateful. Talking to Joanne, however, she showed
no judgement, and simply acknowledged that all of it, from
trying to conceive, through pregnancy and the early years (and
beyond), can pose a threat to our mental health. Whether the
hormones she was subject to as part of her IVF cycle affected
her mood is hard to say, but it is certainly clear she was under
both an emotional and physical onslaught, and unfortunately

during this period was also going through a stressful period at work, which she says "absorbed a significant amount of my physical and emotional time." She talks about a "life-affirming moment" which came after her first round of IVF failed, and she was told she would need to take unpaid leave if she went for another round. She took herself to a park and let go, phoning her mother in tears. Her friends and family rallied, and convinced her to set up her own business, which she believes was a turning point for her. She had one last chance of IVF, with low chances of success due to a low egg count.

At the same time as she finished her job and began her new, self-employed, career, she discovered she was pregnant. The second round of IVF had not only produced a pregnancy, but also three frozen embryos – giving her hope for the family she had always wanted. Although working for herself is less stable financially, with fewer obvious benefits, she is convinced that this step helped the second IVF round towards success. She had a beautiful baby boy, and at the time of writing, she is pregnant with her second child – another boy. She says that while she is anxious about the financial implications of a second child, she loves the flexibility she has and feels that it is important to be a positive role model for her children to grow and to respect women.

"I had longed to become a mum for so many years, yet the length of wait had also allowed me to see some of the parenting challenges my close friends and family faced." She says that whenever her child has been up in the night or simply grizzly, she has found solace in reminding herself how lucky she is to have him. She is convinced that this positive thinking has helped prevent her from becoming too low. For her, motherhood has *more than* matched up to her expectations.

Interestingly, it is now that she is expecting a second child that she feels she is coming back down to earth a bit, because another baby necessitates some practical thinking. But, working through the calculations and possibilities of the coming year, she says simply, "we can do it!"

Despite her very impressive positive outlook, there was one major practical issue which threatened to derail Joanne: feeding. She encountered some fairly extreme views on Facebook groups from people criticising her when she introduced some formula top-ups for her son. I realise the obvious retort to this is "just don't read it", but it is fascinating how compelled people can be, particularly vulnerable people, in situations like that, to return to online abusers again and again. I well remember almost seeking out some of the more extreme breast-feeding views, even though now with hindsight I realise that there are extremists in everything, and they rarely represent the majority. Also, really – who cares? But at the time, in a period where "Breast is best" is resounding around our frazzled little minds, feeding becomes an enormous, emotive obstacle. Fortunately Joanne had, as did I, supportive friends and family and midwives who helped her to see that her son was flourishing, and to have faith in her decisions.

I had seen and dipped into the incredible online PND community. I had not realised, because I was very fortunate in being able to conceive my children relatively easily, that there was the equivalent level of support for those struggling with infertility. Joanne found great comfort from friends she made through Twitter during her experiences. She emphasises that her family and friends, together with these online friends, were an enormous support to her. Some of her childhood friends had lived with chronic mental health issues, so were very conscious of the risk of PND, and they supported Joanne during the newborn period, to try to pre-empt it developing. They also wanted her to know that they would be quick to get her the support she needed, if she had shown signs of developing it. She says she feels very lucky that she did not get it, but she does know others in similar circumstances (i.e. history of infertility) who did, and felt very guilty for feeling that way when they had longed for a child for many years. She knows that some in that situation may not seek help for a long time.

People talk about induction with a degree of dread: there is a general assumption it will be long, drawn out, and often result in some kind of intervention. Actually I have heard several mothers tell a very different story, but unfortunately Joanne is not one of them. At two weeks overdue, she began the induction process. She was in the induction suite for three days, waiting. Inevitably the pressure the staff were under meant that she was deferred repeatedly while they dealt with emergencies.

She is positive about most of the midwives who looked after her, but had one fairly brutal-sounding one who barely let her leave the Tacograph machine to go to the toilet. Her induction followed lines which will be familiar to anyone who has been in an antenatal class and been warned of this... her membrane was broken and a syntocinon drip was given. She took only gas and air for 11 hours of intense contractions, when she found that she had not dilated at all, and accepted an epidural. At this stage both mum and baby were in distress, so an emergency C-section was performed. Despite the situation, she describes the birth itself in very positive terms, with a large, very attentive team caring for her. "No words could ever do justice to how I felt getting the most beautiful little boy... my son... in my arms for the first time. To this day, it is the place I now take myself back to when I want to feel complete bliss. It felt that the whole world (and especially this beautiful baby) was just glowing... though 11 hours of gas and air may have helped with that. Somehow it felt like everything was going to be alright." Unsurprisingly, given this reaction, she feels she bonded immediately with her son, who was a very contented little baby, despite not getting enough milk at first. This blissful state was deflated somewhat by what followed – once again, a mum having to sleep on soiled sheets, and receiving not even the most basic help with baby care. She is philosophical though: "no long-term harm was done". She also remembers being on a ward with other mums who had had emergency C-sections, and the camaraderie she found there. This is such a striking contrast to my own and other PND mothers' experiences that I felt it worth sharing, because it's helpful to remember how it can be.

It was on the post-natal ward though that Joanne's feeding issues started. She was given conflicting advice by many different midwives. One day her latch was deemed "perfect", the next she had her feeding cushion removed, position changed and suddenly her nipples were agonisingly sore. She was refused discharge on the grounds that her baby son had lost too much weight. By this stage, and in spite of her very positive attitude, she started to feel desperate. By using combination feeding they were able to get out of hospital the next day, to her immense relief. Breast-feeding still stands out, nearly two years on, as the main challenge of motherhood. "I felt like a failure when, after three months, I had to give up." Her return to work has been relatively smooth, as much as it can be when running your own business, but she sounds very aware that stress from work is something which can get to her. Working alone means she has no team to share ideas with. However, she sounds very excited and happy about the arrival of her second child. She sums up what she has learnt in the first two years of motherhood:

"There is more than one right way of parenting. Don't allow anyone to pressure you … Not all midwives are experts in breast-feeding – trust your instincts and find professional support that works with you… Don't let any hospital staff push you around. Have a birthing plan, but don't get too hung up on everything going to plan. Be aware of the various birthing experiences and options and be assertive with midwives on what you want from the birthing experience. If you're feeling down – it's OK, you're not alone and you're still a great mum. Talk to someone you trust, engage with support groups (in person or online if you prefer). Ask for help if you need it. That is ok too. Don't allow the pressures to take away from the enjoyment of being a parent. Try to still set aside a little time for yourself – whether it's watching a film, reading a book, having a meal with friends (or if you can get willing babysitters, your partner)."

She then adds: "That's probably already too much advice – basically go with the flow, seek support when needed and don't put too much pressure on yourself to do everything perfectly."

18

Location, location – isolation and motherhood

Melissa's story

A lot of the women I speak to mention the role their partner plays in their recovery from PND. But what about the ones who don't have a partner – or who do, and a supportive one at that, but for whatever reason he/she is unable to help much on a practical level. I imagine this might be the case for, say, a military wife. And then I spoke to Melissa, whose husband has a long-term debilitating illness, as well as a demanding job. Her first child was born when they were living in a very rural and isolated area where they knew few people. She explains that she hadn't really given much thought to what motherhood would be like. She found the experience shocking right from the start, when she had a C-section she had never envisaged. She had very little support in place. Her friends were a long way away, family could not or would not help. There was a succession of midwives, doctors and health visitors but the care sounds inconsistent. The birth itself, she says, was "Traumatic! After a false alarm [I] got sent home from Birthing Centre, was back 24 hours later. Had a bob in the birthing pool, waters broken manually, then ambulance transfer... not nice, unhelpful midwife at Maternity Unit, epidural which was then topped up for an emergency C-Section, when it was apparent [the baby] was stuck." Despite this start, she does feel that the bond with her son was instant. After a four day stay in the hospital, mother and son returned home. The hospital stay was difficult – unable to move much after her C-section, and in a room on her own, Melissa found it hard to care for her new baby. She was reliant on staff. Back at home, the first two weeks were terrible: "looking back it was just 'black'". It was winter, the baby was struggling to put on weight, screamed after each feed, developed bad nappy rash and then started to lose weight. After his two weeks' paternity leave, Melissa's husband had to go back to work, leaving her solely reliant on the Health Visitor, who unfortunately was not especially supportive. Four weeks in, the family ended up in hospital twice and she ended up on a lactose-free diet. She explains that this was particularly challenging in a very rural area, trying to obtain the food she needed to maintain the diet. Eventually she began topping the baby up and using infant Gaviscon and Infacol. Lack of sleep and a lack of sufficient outside help mean Melissa struggled on until he was 12 weeks, until she realised "he really wasn't getting anything from me at all!"

I felt very sad hearing Melissa's story because, like so many, just getting a diagnosis, let alone follow up help, sounds like it was very difficult. In her case, matters were complicated by the fact her husband has a chronic illness which mean he was very limited in how much he could help. She tells me that as far as she knows there is no support for families in this situation.

"I thought I was doing ok. At my six-week check and first venture out of the house by myself after the C-Section, the doctor asked me various questions and actually said that she was trying to make me cry to see if I was post-natal. Even after a telephone consult with the Psych team at hospital, I could not be prescribed any anti-depressants "(She isn't sure whether that was due to breast-feeding or the lactose-free diet she had been put on). She was referred to the Mental Health Team, where she had an assessment appointment after another six weeks when her son was 12 weeks old. "I had spent time telling the female assessor that [my husband] was not in good health himself and often in hospital or away with work, when home was exhausted so in bed really early due to his health issues. I also told her that I had no family help, my parents – for reasons best known to themselves - weren't overly interested in helping in any way, relations having broken down. She then spent quite a while telling me that [my husband] must do the 10pm feed and that I had to pull myself together. I left devastated, having wasted an hour of my life."

A second assessment led to a diagnosis of mild depression. By this point she had stopped breast-feeding and so felt able to take a course of anti-depressants. This is an interesting point, because four years later when I started my first course of anti-depressants it was made very clear to me that it is entirely possible to breast-feed on certain drugs. It made me think that, once again, Melissa lost out just because of where she was living and the care she was able to access at the time.

As well as medication, she had counselling for over a year. Meanwhile life was still very tough. She talks about the daily challenge of keeping on top of everything. They had decided to use washable nappies. However it was winter in rural Wales and, combined with a sick baby and a husband exhausted by his illness and work, this added up to "loss of marbles!"

A friend who visited when her son was about seven months old advised her to do no more than one household chore a day (which seems like excellent advice). She thinks it was about then that the family moved to disposable nappies too.

"Everything seemed like a real challenge... I didn't know what I was doing with (her son), I didn't understand why he cried constantly as a new baby." The constant crying was actually due to lactose intolerance, but this can be very tricky, and slow, to diagnose. In the meantime Melissa persevered. She is one of many mothers I've spoken to for whom feeding seems to be at the heart of their depression story. The hinterland issues – the fact she had moved away from family and friends in the previous year, followed by a difficult birth – compounded matters. She says herself she's not surprised "it was all so black". Despite her experience, she went on to have two more children. She didn't suffer to the same degree after her second, but did with her third child, a summer baby who struggled to gain weight. Now living in a different area, she was prescribed anti-depressants which she is still taking three and a half years later. I was interested in how Melissa found having subsequent children, particularly the logistics of juggling them. She explained that emotionally she had concerns about having a daughter due to a difficult relationship with her own mother. She was also worried about having a second C-section, which she ended up having. She says, very honestly, that as a result for the first day or two she felt "really cross" with her little girl but quickly got over that feeling, and thinks that having had her in Spring perhaps helped with her mood: "I didn't quite feel so lost." Having moved areas and made some friends there, she also felt much more settled and comfortable generally. Her oldest child was almost three and a half by the time she had her second, and she explains that she had taught him to be fairly self-sufficient by then, a pattern which she repeated with her second, after she had her third child. Although she has moved on from the PND experience, her day-to-day life is still a struggle – the logistics of three small children and a husband with ill-health take their toll. Again, very honestly, she admits that despite always wanting a big family, "three was stretching me a little too far" – and they certainly won't be having any more.

Melissa is surely an example of someone who fell foul of the postcode lottery picture which has emerged of perinatal mental health care across the country. By moving between having her first and second children, she had deeply contrasting experiences. She says that she believes partners "should be encouraged to contact the doctor or health visitor if the mother isn't doing so well so to access help. I'm a good liar when it comes to feelings, so the health visitor wouldn't necessarily know if I wasn't doing well – particularly if there is no continuity of care." Her other conclusion from her experience is that the breast-feeding policy was a big obstacle to her recovery. "I then wished to be fair with each of the children so put myself through the trauma of insisting that I would feed each myself for 12 weeks before I gave up." This appears to have worked with the second child, but Melissa's youngest, like her oldest, had feeding issues. She also comments that it did not feel to her as though there was much support available to mums like her, with one parent battling a debilitating chronic illness.

19

Feeding issues – them and us

Julia's story

Julia is 41, and had postnatal depression – diagnosed four months in – after her first child was born in 2004. Hearing her story made me think about what has changed in the decade or more since her experience.

When talking about what her preconceptions of motherhood were, Julia references her own mother a lot. "My mother had always brought me up to believe that motherhood was something that you just did and got on with, that giving birth was fine and women who screamed or thought childbirth was painful were weak. I assumed that I would breast-feed no problem, that we would bond straight away, that it would be tiring but worth every moment."

Julia is not the only woman I have spoken to who said this about her own mother's perspective. My own mum also used to say, after watching Channel 4's "One Born Every Minute", that she couldn't understand all these women making such a big fuss. I wonder if part of this though is the selective memory we all fall prey to after giving birth? And also if part of it is a protectiveness towards our own children – almost wanting to convince yourself and them that it won't be painful.

In Julia's case, she reflects that she was fortunate: "I think my body took itself to the limit of what it could do and I managed to pop them out fine – just luck nothing else, no super powers, or feeling of superiority over anyone else who found it far harder." This is a really refreshing comment to hear, as someone who found birth very difficult. She even calls her first birth "enjoyable, bizarrely". She had planned a water birth but once things got going did not want to move from the bed. She does comment that she wished she'd been warned that she might lose control of her bodily functions in childbirth – particularly vomiting, which was a real shock and came as she was pushing.

However it was the bit which came next which Julia struggled with. "Breast-feeding was a nightmare, my daughter had gastric reflux and I didn't sleep for four days. It was a very challenging start." I can relate to the reflux and feeding issues only too well, and I was going through them several years down the line – my feeling is that reflux is more widely understood now. The problems with feeding seemed to stem from a poor latch, which led to a lesion on one breast, in turn bringing on two separate bad bouts of mastitis. She was made to feel that the poor latch was her fault. She links this to her feeling that she didn't bond with her daughter straightaway "although she was gorgeous... that feeling of overwhelming love wasn't there right at the start and took a very long time to come." A three day stay in hospital with no sleep, rest or assistance and a baby who would not feed, and was vomiting feeds, compounded this feeling.

On going home, she had the support of her husband during his two weeks of paternity leave: "an absolute rock", and various midwives, "none of whom were particularly supportive". Her mum was very helpful but the couple lived away from their families, so there was a limit to the support they could have. She describes the first few weeks as "pretty horrendous. She wouldn't latch on, slept all the time and we battled to wake her to feed. She threw everything up that we managed to get inside her, but the midwives and then health visitor didn't accept she might have reflux because she was a little girl who was born bang on time. The emphasis was firmly on breast-feeding and I was told I must not bottle-feed at all - so, because my daughter would not latch on, I had to express. The midwives and health visitor insisted that I tried to get her to latch on every three hours, on the dot. I did this and would fail for about half an hour, when I would then feed her expressed milk, which she would then throw up. This whole process would take about an hour and a half and would then need to be repeated an hour and a half later, 24 hours a day. I had to set my alarm clock to go off in the night and of course had then to express and wash and sterilise in between. This went on for five weeks, even after a gastric reflux diagnosis, two horrendous bouts of mastitis with fever and hallucinations and my daughter being admitted into hospital as she went into shock and began to shut down."

Unsurprisingly, this all led to a breakdown about four months in. "I finally hit the wall and slid down." Julia and her husband saw the GP together and she was given Prozac. Arrangements were made for a mental health nurse to visit her, which never happened. Fortunately, she returned to work a month later, which she credits with saving her, and making her feel as though she didn't need the anti-depressants. She stayed on them for six months and says she hasn't looked back, but does think it's worrying that there was no follow-up. A good support network got her through, although her mother was "of the generation where you just get on with it, and I think slightly ashamed of this 'weakness' I had shown".

Julia remarks that her antenatal classes contained no suggestion that breast-feeding might be anything other than straightforward. As a result, she found this side of things – and the resultant lack of bonding – the biggest challenge. Her classes didn't cover the possibility of bottle-feeding (or the practicalities) – which seems to be a common experience. I remember posting to this effect on a forum when Joe was little, only to have someone remark, "Well how hard can it be to make up a bottle?". Actually, given the strain new mothers are already under, and the changing advice about how to prepare bottles safely, it can be very hard indeed. That's not even touching the emotional issues. Julia talks about feeling crippled by the "guilt associated with 'failing' to feed my daughter". She felt so exhausted that it was a struggle to think through even the simplest of tasks. The feeling of isolation, and the complete change of lifestyle took its toll.

It's gratifying to hear that, despite this start, she was able to enjoy watching her little girl grow – and now they have a wonderful relationship. Once the depression departed, she felt able to properly bond with her daughter. Her second birth, as with her first, was good and she felt more prepared in any case. "The bonding was there straightaway with my little boy and it was love at first sight. I decided to try again with breast-feeding, because I loved the idea of the ease of it, no washing and sterilising, and quietly got on with it, although I was prepared for it not working this time (I even bought a large tub of formula from Tesco on the way home from the hospital, just in case!)."

She thinks that being more relaxed second time around, and possibly being distracted by having a toddler to look after, it was all a bit easier. "We were allowed to leave the hospital just hours after he was born because I couldn't bear the idea of staying in again - I was still as exhausted, but at least I was at home and knackered, with my husband and daughter there and cups of tea and toys and the telly where necessary!" The three year age gap seemed to work well, and she found her second child an easy baby who fed and slept without problem. She even says she "almost" found it easier with two. She does say though that two children are enough: "I never want to feel like that again and so am acutely aware of any familiar feelings of depression or feeling down - I choose to tackle these head on now and take action to prevent it getting any worse, and so far this has worked for me. I know not to ignore these signs and make sure I talk to someone about it, make sure I keep myself occupied, however hard that might be." Her advice to others going through something similar is : "Listen to yourself, make your own choices and keep talking about everything. Don't alter your parenting style to please or impress other people and if you feel down, don't shy away from it, talk to someone and don't feel ashamed, ever. You do get through it - but you will need help, and you need that help for your children."

20

The ties that bond: depressed mums can and do bond

Sophie's story

Sophie is 39, and had her son in 2009. She says she wasn't the type of girl who grows up wanting children. "I had expected not to have children in truth, so I didn't have a fixed image of what it would be like." She thinks she had envisaged herself as more carefree, more of a 'hippy' mum than she turned out to be. One of the things that really strikes me about Sophie's story is that she appears to have bonded with her son very early and very strongly. "I didn't realise how profoundly I would feel for my child. I bought a sling before he was born imagining that if he was crying I would put him in a sling and get on with washing up or tidying. In fact if he was crying I couldn't do anything but hold him as it broke my heart." She wrote to me describing a feeling of being "blown away" by the love she felt for him – though this was coupled with an enormous and ongoing sense of guilt, constantly querying whether she was doing the right thing for him. This, she is sure, "will always be there." When I met Sophie, she talked about this a bit more, explaining that her son is still very connected to her, and it sounds as though he has always picked up on her moods, so that when she began to feel depressed when he was around two months old, she felt his feeding was immediately affected.

The possibility of getting PND was definitely something that occurred to Sophie before having her son, partly because a family friend had suffered from puerperal psychosis. She describes feeling anxious about being isolated. But what actually happened was that she didn't feel alone at all – she made good friends, and found the local health centre and children's centre very supportive. Family were not nearby, but Sophie doesn't think this is necessarily negative, as it meant she had to get on with things herself, and was able to do so without being observed. What happened instead was that Sophie became anxious. "I felt sick and this made me more anxious, as I was worried about what would happen to him if I did become sick, though coupled with this did fantasise about being hospitalised and someone else having to take over and me being less responsible."

Hearing this took me back to Joe being around four weeks old. He had a complex health issue – an ulcerated haemangioma – which necessitated a visit to A&E late one night. I remember thinking, what if he's kept in overnight? And part of me, not a small part either, hoped that perhaps he would be, so that for 12 hours I would have both sleep and a complete absence of responsibility.

Sophie's birth was a long one, following induction. She describes it as "exhausting... shocking and surreal", a feeling not helped by the gas and air which made her feel "outside myself... there was a heart monitor on the baby, the sound of which drove me a bit crazy." Despite the long "bloody awful endless birth", her first words on her son's delivery were "it was worth it" – she felt the rush of love straightaway. Like my experience with my first son, Sophie was kept in hospital for a week because her son had jaundice. She talks about the box (phototherapy) which was meant to help with the baby's jaundice, but she found it hard to keep him in it, and would take him out to feed him and hold him. They were given a billy blanket in the end. I found this anecdote a really interesting illustration of the way Sophie bonded straightaway with her son. When Joe was 'under the light', I felt much the same relief I would anticipate a few weeks later at the thought of him being kept in hospital overnight. The warmth meant that for once he was not crying when he was laid down. It was the one time during a week's hospital stay that I had any sleep. It would never have occurred to me to take him out (partly because I took all the directions from staff absolutely literally). I did like that we could stroke him through the holes in the side of the box, but I didn't feel a strong urge to take him out. I was very worried that the little 'sunglasses' they had given him to protect his eyes were slipping down and would leave his eyes vulnerable to damage, and I would constantly tweak them.

Talking to Sophie, we reminisced about those awkward days on a post-natal ward when you need to do things away from your baby – go to the loo, take a shower. I confided that I had felt very guilty years after Joe's birth, when I realised I never thought twice about leaving him. I would just go off and have a shower! This was despite the fact he used to scream a lot. I only really thought about this when I heard someone talking about how difficult it had been to get the hospital crib's wheels to work so they could wheel the baby to the bathroom with them. I had one of those "Is it just me?" moments. Talking to Sophie, I was quite relieved, given her obvious immediate bond with her son, when she said, "well what else could we do?! We had to leave them to go to the toilet!" It still saddens me though when I think back to those first few hours; whenever the community midwife who had been there for Joe's delivery checked in on me she would chide me for not holding him. She was clearly anxious about feeding. I was exhausted and totally strung out with tiredness. It just didn't occur to me to pick him up. One of the first pictures, if not the first picture, of us both shows me on the phone and Joe lying in the crib next to me. It still makes my heart catch a bit thinking about that. A few weeks later, by now back at home, I had a similar moment with a playmat. I had laid Joe on the mat, not really thinking about the fact it was very thin and we had solid wooden floorboards. My friend said gently, "Do you have a blanket or anything to soften the surface, just for his head?" I was startled; I hadn't even thought. Second time around, with Ted, the bond was there far quicker, and I did feel I was thinking more "like a mum", although I would still question myself at any opportunity.

For Sophie, it sounds as though the anxiety kicked in quite a few weeks later – more than ten weeks in. She talks about the relief of getting home after her week in hospital. She says it felt peaceful being at home, though of course she had bad days. There were logistical issues, such as getting in and out of her flat with a pushchair and negotiating public transport for hospital appointments. "I was very tired, and worried about if I was doing the right thing, but in other ways felt I could do anything and I often think did too much and should perhaps have done less... but I felt like I needed to get out." She highlights the sense of responsibility and the sheer domestic drudgery of motherhood as the areas she found toughest. Possibly uniquely among the mothers I've spoken to, Sophie thinks that being a mum allowed her to be more herself than being at work ever had. The shared experience with others, and resulting friendships, has been an enjoyable side. Sophie stopped working, and instead pursued her studies for a period, giving her more time for her son. She has since changed her line of work, and feels she has made "a new start of sorts". She talks enthusiastically of the life she shares with her son, and it's clear she enjoys it: "I enjoy the life I have with my child, I love his curiosity, and in a sense learning new information with him, the loving relationship that we have with each other."

Sophie told me that about ten weeks in she was diagnosed with post-natal depression. She was under the care of a very supportive GP who saw her at least once a week to check on her; "she made a huge difference to my experience." With the GP's support Sophie took the decision to go onto anti-depressants (Sertraline), which she estimates took about four weeks to help her to feel like she could cope. She was referred to a local support group, which met weekly, and which was partly social but also included some CBT. Because of her previous worries about being isolated, Sophie was very proactive about joining groups and building a network of friends. Her experience was that the free groups felt less judgemental, more inclusive. She was also seen by a post-partum psychologist twice.

I was intrigued by Sophie's fairly fleeting reference to "feeling sick" as she initially gave little other detail about her depressive symptoms when we spoke. Having met up with her to talk through her story further, I got the impression she is a very positive person. So a lot of what she initially told me was the "good stuff" – the instant bonding, the pleasure in making new friends. I wanted to know more about the bad stuff – what did she mean about thinking she might be hospitalised? We met up, and Sophie told me, "I thought I was ill." Around eight weeks in, she took several trips which in retrospect she thinks stretched her too far. The last one was down to the South West, to see her mother – a long journey, coupled with solo care of her baby for a few days, in the sense that her boyfriend wasn't there to help. Although it's clear she sees this trip as the catalyst, she does reflect that actually PND was probably coming, but she hadn't noticed it at the time. She explains that because she felt unable to let her baby cry for even a moment, long car journeys were incredibly stressful, with many, many stops. The final straw appears to have been during her visit to her mum's, when she returned from a brief solo trip to the shops to buy nappies to find her baby crying uncontrollably. For someone who found it agonising to hear her child cry at all, I can imagine how much of a trigger this was. As a result, Sophie became more and more anxious, to the point where she couldn't eat, and at the same time was experiencing frequent vomiting and diarrhoea. She didn't realise at first that these might be symptoms of her anxiety. We talk about people being "worried sick" but few of us realise that anxiety can have such a dramatic bodily response.

Sophie became convinced that she was ill. She asked her boyfriend to come and collect her and the baby, as the thought of a long train journey back home with him was far too daunting. Sophie was sent for a series of hospital tests, which were all negative. She talks about this as confirmation that it was in her head, but says it was actually quite helpful to know this, and to start taking the appropriate action. She was given the option of anti-depressants, and although her GP said she could probably manage without them, after a couple of days to consider it, Sophie opted to start them. Sophie sounds very matter of fact about the diagnosis; she found it helpful, and it enabled her to start to feel better. This makes sense, particularly when she tells me about various points when it felt like someone else "took charge" – for example her aunt taking her to the hospital for all her tests. I can remember feeling similarly, that I just wanted someone to come along and take control for me.

The anti-depressant had side effects – which were both good and bad. Diarrhoea was one, but Sophie was used to this from her anxiety-related symptoms. And it stimulated her appetite, but since one of the effects of being anxious was that she had lost her appetite, Sophie saw this is a very helpful thing. In any case, after a few weeks, the side effects settled, and she remained on the medication for about a year.

When things were at their worst, Sophie said her low point was 10am. This was a time when her baby would be grizzly, but also when she would be throwing up. However, the anti-depressants worked: she began to feel better relatively quickly. I was curious as to whether she had told people what was happening, and she said generally she did, and one friend she made when her baby was very young says that, knowing her now, i.e. not depressed, she can see how obvious it was she was depressed. But of course, generally, those friends we make only after or just before the birth of our children don't know the "real" us, so it can be hard to admit that there is something wrong. Sophie also told me an anecdote about bumping into her neighbour – also a mother – and being asked how she was. Sophie had been on the verge of saying, "I'm fine" when her own mother, who was with her at the time, caught her eye and encouraged her to tell the truth, which she did. As a result the neighbour immediately invited her to come for tea the next day – crucially setting a time for it, which, as Sophie says, was very effective at convincing her to go. From the women I've spoken to, a picture starts to emerge of not necessarily one stand-out panacea for PND, but a host of small, simple gestures, moments which may seem completely ordinary to the world at large, but to the woman lost in the mist, they add up to the sum of the parts which spell recovery. Sophie also made a very interesting point about telling people: that in doing so, it helped her to feel secure – the more people who knew, the more she felt there was a strong safety net there. That seems to me to be very important. The obvious advice we give to people with depression is "tell someone", but that shouldn't just be because it's good to talk. There is a safety point too, because depression is dangerous, and of course without help, without people knowing, it's an illness that can be fatal.

Sophie was assessed by a psychiatrist, she thinks to check her bond with her baby. Of all the people I talked to, she is one of the few who says she had that bond very strongly, right from the start. But her mentioning this need for her doctor to check it was there, reminded me of how often I was asked this by well-meaning GPs and midwives in the early days. "How's the bonding?" it seemed to me then, as it still does now, an incredibly inane question, and one which makes it very obvious what the 'right' answer is. Whenever I was asked it, I would lie – which I didn't generally do about PND. I suspect in part this was because I was afraid to really study my relationship with my baby at that stage. The bond was there, but it was fragile, and like my son when he was in utero, it was not growing at the expected rate.

Sophie talks a lot about her very supportive GP, and the many kind and helpful midwives and health visitors she met during that low period. Her GP saw her every week over a long time, often just for five minutes, but it was enough to reassure them both that Sophie was doing well – and that if she wasn't, there was her safety net again. The GP very sensibly scheduled Sophie's appointments for the time of the week when she knew things might be a bit tougher, pacing her week for her so that for instance she'd have just started to feel low a few days after the weekend or a visit from her mum, but would have the appointment to hold on to. I had forgotten, but my own GP did something similar with me.

Sophie told me that she found reflecting on her experience of PND difficult, more so, I think, than she had expected to. Having had post-natal depression is one (although not the main) reason why she decided not to have any more children. "I do think I want to avoid that risk especially as I wouldn't want to be in that state for my current family." She recalls her doctor telling her at the time that even if she was crying, she should not avoid holding her baby because it could actually be more damaging not to hold the baby (I must say I'm not entirely sure of the wisdom of this advice, I know if it had been given to me I'd have immediately worried about whether I'd damaged Joe by not holding him enough). The point for Sophie is that this makes her wonder how it would be for an older child if she was to go through depression again. It's certainly something which has crossed my mind when considering more children.

Sophie's advice to others: "I tell them to be kind to themselves, that it is exhausting and to not try to do too much but also that it is amazing and that I was blown away by the fact that I could feel so much love. I also say to build networks around them so that they have people in place before the bad day comes to act as a safety net."

21

The in-patient: when a mother is hospitalised

Lindsey's story

In October 2014, to mark World Mental Health Day, I co-ordinated a tweet chat with the Maudsley Hospital in London and my client, Brixton Live – an alliance of cultural organisations based in Brixton in South London. We decided to focus on post-natal depression, in part because many of Brixton Live's members work with families in the community, and we felt it was an issue that affected many of them. The Maudsley brought in psychiatric nurses from their residential Mother and Baby Unit, Bethlem, based in Kent. These nurses took part in the tweet chat, fielding questions – including the perennial "will my child be taken away from me?" with skill and reassurance. It was the first time I really became aware of these residential units, and I concluded that it would be helpful to hear from a woman who had been an in-patient as a result of PND. By chance, a relative had a friend who had stayed in a similar unit in another county, and she put us in touch. Initially, and understandably, Lindsey was nervous about taking part; her experience had clearly been severe, and felt very much in her past, as it had happened seven years ago. We decided to talk on the phone and take it slowly. Once we started talking though, her story came quite freely. Her daughter is now seven, and she said to me that though occasionally she thinks about counselling, she mostly just feels she has moved on to other things. As her story unfolded, it became evident that the bumpy start she had had, experiencing severe depression, had been superseded by more present concerns: her daughter has ongoing medical problems.

I asked her to talk me through her pregnancy and birth initially. She started by saying her pregnancy had been straightforward, and that her mood was good throughout – this was very positive, in the context of a history of anxiety. However, she did suffer from extreme morning sickness. I asked if this was hyperemesis. She said it was probably a borderline case, but, as she never needed intervention, it was never diagnosed as such. The outcome though, was that she lost weight, which she now thinks in retrospect contributed to her post-natal mood, perhaps as a result of the hormone changes taking place. Despite the extreme sickness, she found pregnancy quite enjoyable. She planned to give birth at home, and things began well, but ultimately took so long, and there was concern that the baby was struggling, that she was transferred – via ambulance – to hospital to receive "the full works". From there a familiar pattern developed; epidural, attempted ventouse and finally forceps. Lindsey describes the process as "fairly traumatic... I felt like I was on a different planet." And throughout, her husband was present, and very frightened by what was happening. At this we both paused and reflected that perhaps dads are overlooked too often in this picture. Mums are, quite rightly, the focus. But perhaps there is a tendency to play down how traumatic watching your partner go through a difficult birth (or indeed, any birth), can be.

My own experience of antenatal classes was that the men in the group were patronised, and almost mocked for not knowing for example that women would need maternity pads after the birth, and they would be in charge of buying them. I understand the focus has to be on preparing the mum for her birth in any antenatal class, but it might be helpful if their partners have some preparation for what they may be about to witness. NCT provided Lindsey with a good group of friends, and she says that PND was certainly mentioned, though not in great depth. Her generalised anxiety, a feature of her pre-pregnancy life, seemed to recede in pregnancy, but she was very aware that she might be a candidate for PND given her history, and to prepare for this she and her husband discussed what they would do. She remembers telling him to make her go to the doctor if he saw the signs. Remembering my conversation with Dr Lang at Tommy's, I asked her how proactive she found her doctor and midwife during the pregnancy in asking her about her mental health. She thought they probably had not been proactive, and she felt she herself had not been because her anxiety at that stage felt negligible; it didn't seem worth mentioning her past. She also said, confirming what every healthcare professional has said to me, that the fear of not saying the right thing was always present.

Back in the labour ward, Lindsey's baby arrived and she felt immediately "wrong… I had her in my arms, I felt traumatised, disconnected, no rush of love… a wave of anxiety." This completely took her aback. She had a strong sense that this was not how she was supposed to feel. Hindsight has helped her to piece together some of the puzzle. Exhaustion after a long and difficult labour, her weight loss, the birth itself and possibly her history are surely all contributing factors to her state of mind post partum. On top of this, her husband had to go home for the night, as partners being allowed to stay overnight was not hospital policy. The description she gives of how she felt at that point brought back strong memories of my first night in hospital after Joe's birth. Lindsey was already terrified: she felt disabled by anxiety, and as though she couldn't look after her baby. She struggled with breast-feeding, and, on a practical level, was lying in sheets which needed to be changed (I thought to myself grimly this clearly wasn't something that had only happened to me). She remembers crying constantly, and keeping her curtains closed. I could picture this, because it's exactly what I did. I still find it strange when people reminisce about the camaraderie on the post-natal ward: I didn't even register the other women's faces. But where Ben and I were thwarted in our half-crazed attempt to discharge ourselves from hospital, Lindsey, fatefully, was successful. Looking back, cannot believe she was allowed to go. But she was, and she now knows she really was not well enough to leave hospital that day. She felt very strongly that she would be alright at home, a feeling I can empathise with. But of course, she was not: at home, things felt just as bad, and, after two days of pretending, she had to concede she needed help.

She had found herself unable to sleep, plagued by nightmares, which, on top of being exhausted post partum, took their toll. Her midwife was somewhat surprised when Lindsey told her very directly that she had PND. I have found too, that early awareness is sometimes not taken seriously. There is a perception that it can only kick in after six weeks or some other arbitrary starting point. Perhaps Lindsey's experience of mental health problems helped her self-awareness. Fortunately the midwife was clearly convinced enough to summon help, in the form of a mental health crisis team. She began a series of different medications and appointments. She became fixated on imagined problems, convincing herself that her baby only cried when she saw her mother, but was alright for everyone else. She couldn't breast-feed, and at one point was given sedatives so fairly early on her husband took on the job of feeding their new baby. "He was the mum... I was too terrified, when I heard her cry I felt really anxious." Hearing this, I felt relieved for her that in a catalogue of obstacles which added up to a very difficult start, she was not pushed to breastfeed at the expense of her mental health.

However, despite this small mercy, and the involvement of the specialists, the grip of post-natal depression was too strong. Very honestly – both then, and now in telling me – Lindsey says that she reached a point where she did not feel safe around her daughter. She was worried she would harm her. She immediately told her husband, who took her to the GP for help. The first approach they took was to put her onto a mental health ward, which she said was understandably scary. Worse, her daughter was not with her – she was allowed to visit only, not to stay with her. After two or three weeks, her sister intervened. She was moved to a Mother and Baby Unit about an hour's drive away from her home. She describes how, on arrival here, she had an initial feeling of relief as the staff took complete care of the baby, then slowly helped her to build up a routine, taking on more of her daughter's care, one night feed at a time. I was impressed. I told her it sounded like a really positive environment. It wasn't quite so simple though. She told me that following the initial relief, she plummeted into a deep depression, as she was made to do everything under the staff's watch: taking a bath with someone in the room, wondering if she would ever get out. She was there for three months. Her medication was revised, and she attended a weekly meeting with all the professionals involved in her case, which she says could be terrifying. These were the people who had the power over her freedom: whether she would be trusted with more time on her own (privileges, in a sense), or whether she continued to need supervision. Despite the close bonds women developed in the unit, the results of these meetings could cause difficult emotions for them as they watched their peers gain more freedom not always matched by their own progress. The women sounded very protective, looking out for new patients, helping each other out.

Throughout all this, Lindsey's husband –while working full-time – travelled to visit his wife and daughter almost every day and at every weekend. It sounds as though this was bittersweet, because at the end of each visit of course she had to say goodbye again. I asked how her relationship with her daughter was developing, in the midst of all this. "She didn't feel real... she felt very disjointed from me, and the relationship took a while." A psychiatrist who Lindsey was seeing reassured her that this was normal, and was her anxiety manifesting itself. Gradually, she took charge of her daughter more and more, though the unit ensured there was never any pressure on her to do so. She feels fortunate to have had the care of a very skilled perinatal psychiatrist's care throughout her stay. When she did leave the unit, she was on a lot of medications, which she gradually came off under the supervision of a general psychiatrist, who she says frankly "didn't have a clue" about perinatal mental health. Lithium worked well for her, and slowly she stripped back her other medications. She continued to see the psychiatrist for another three or four months. She felt she had come out the other side. Sadly her difficulties did not end there. Firstly, there was the guilt: a family member was initially angry with her, suggesting that she had somehow let the PND happen by not addressing her previous anxiety. Yet one of the things which really struck me on hearing Lindsey's story is that, unlike so many women who find it incredibly hard to admit to having PND, she was honest with herself, her husband and her midwife right from the start. I say this to her, and she simply says, "I couldn't have not told them... I felt suicidal." She is affected by any story about new mums who have severe PND, particularly media stories about mums who go missing, or kill themselves and their children. "It gets to you... it could have been us." She thinks that we all underestimate the power of hormones perinatally, which is a message I heard from the professionals I talked to, too.

But secondly, and with far greater impact, her daughter became ill almost immediately after she had regained her own mental health. In the years since, the family have had an incredibly challenging time. Her daughter's medical problems have led to a major operation, and a special school. Throughout all this, she says, she hasn't needed any further psychiatric help. I find that astonishing – and perhaps it backs up her theory about perinatal hormones. Her experience at the start of her daughter's life has left her even more conscious of her state of mind. She says that both she and her husband have had wobbly moments, of course, but that they are acutely aware of these and the need to bring things into the open, to talk through problems. "I've learned from PND to be very mindful of the wobbles."

22

When PND is not PND – Psychosis

Blogger Tracey Robinson's story

Often when people think about PND, if they have not had direct experience of it, it is actually the stories of women with post-partum psychosis they are thinking about. Those are the ones which can hit the media, which stay in the mind – although the chances of having it are relatively slim. While more people are sharing their experiences of PND, psychosis can still be seen as a taboo. It's frightening, because we don't understand it. I came across a blog – A Mummy Recovered - by Tracey Robinson, an NHS programme manager and mental health occupational therapist who is also a survivor of both PND and post-partum psychosis. She is very active now on Twitter in the #PND community there. Her first blog entry, "Manic Mummy – my descent into post-partum psychosis", narrates her experience of psychosis in particular.

"Manic Mummy – my descent into post-partum psychosis
Posted on 02/11/2014
by amummyrecovered

So, why am I here writing my first ever blog post? The crux of it is that 10 years ago I suffered from postpartum psychosis, then 6 years ago I suffered from postnatal depression, and until recently I haven't shared my experiences as widely and honestly as I could have done. Sure, I've sometimes spoken about it to certain friends and family who have a good understanding of such things, but I've totally avoided the topic with many others. I occasionally tell my story at training days for professionals, but mostly in my day-to-day home and work life I've buried that part of my history, and tried to move on in a kind of semi-denial that it really happened to me. It's mainly been a self stigmatisation thing.......It's also decidedly painful, and sometimes embarassing, to relive some parts of my experience, and I haven't always felt strong enough to face it. But a few months ago, due to some reactions I got when I told my story, I felt compelled to do it more. I hope that by being open and honest I can contribute to tackling stigma, improving understanding, and offering hope to others. More selfishly I've also finally realised that facing the memories and truths that I've avoided hold the key to me regaining a fully intact self esteem, and saying a final goodbye to the guilt, shame and self blame that still impact on me.

In early 2004 I was a happy expectant mother, looking forward to having a paid 6 months off my career to look after my first baby. Oh how naive I was, as I joyfully engaged in baby showers, and read all the books and magazines about how wonderful new motherhood would be for me! I'd followed all the guidance on how to prepare, and through my rose tinted spectacles I imagined I'd cope just fine because I'd planned for baby's arrival with great precision – an approach that had pulled me pretty successfully through most of life's challenges up until then. But the moment my baby boy was born my dreams of how it would be came crashing down. In fact, it started during the birth itself. Whilst I didn't suffer what would be called a traumatic or medically risky labour I felt totally horrified and overwhelmed by the pain, the indignity and the lack of control I felt over my body. When the worst of that was over and my baby was handed to me I didn't experience the rush of love I was expecting, I just felt panic that despite my tiredness, my pain and the gory mess all around me I still had to take responsibility for this tiny pink creature. At that moment I just wanted him taken away for a while, so I could rest until I felt more ready to cope. But I knew that wasn't what I ought to say, I knew that skin to skin contact and early breast-feeding were really important, and I wanted to get my dream back on track, so I held him and tried to do what the books had recommended. That was huge disappointment number two – he couldn't feed and I really resented myself for that perceived failure to get him off to the best start. Thus followed an exhausting three days and nights in a maternity ward, trying repeatedly to get him to breast-feed with very little support from the staff. As for sleep, it totally eluded me that first night after I'd arrived on the ward at 2am, and with the hustle of the daily ward routines and trying to feed during the night there was little opportunity to properly rest as the days went on. I'd never been so exhausted in my life, I was feeling increasingly emotional and desperately craved sleep. I desperately wanted to get home to my own bed, but they wouldn't let me go until feeding was established. Ultimately

I got myself discharged by saying I'd bottle feed instead, but I was secretly determined to carry on trying to breast-feed as soon as I got home, because I was not prepared to accept failing at that, and because despite not having an intense emotional bond I still felt protective towards my son, and responsible for his future health. I don't know at which point I started to go mad. Maybe it was in the hospital when I had a shower and I was so convinced I heard my baby crying that I opened the door and checked 3 times, only to find him lying fast asleep? Was that an auditory hallucination or just tiredness combined with parental protectiveness? Was my inability to sleep in the hospital a cause or a symptom of the upcoming mania which I would experience? And when we welcomed far too many visitors into our home in the early days, did the continuing lack of rest send me manic, or was I inviting them all because I was already losing a grip on what my priorities should have been? What I do know is that during the first two or three weeks of my son's life my emotions and behavior became increasingly unlike my usual self, and my family and friends got more and more worried about me. At first I was concerned myself, mainly about tiredness. I desperately craved sleep, and I was tearful and panicky every time sleep eluded me, due to either my increasingly active mind, or to feeding issues (I was still trying to breast-feed, with very little improvement and a very hungry baby.) Then came the hallucinations where I would see my baby's head on my husband and on passers by, in place of their own faces. These bizarre experiences distressed and confused me but I assumed them to be products of sleep deprivation combined with normal motherly obsessions with her own baby, so I didn't mention them to anybody. At some point I stopped being worried about lack of sleep, I was in such a manic state that all I experienced was unadulterated happiness. I believed that people who were concerned about me just couldn't recognise that becoming a mother had changed me for the better into a totally positive and carefree person. As my grip on reality loosened I developed false beliefs that we were financially very well off, and I started spending money that we didn't have. As I was totally unable to sleep by then I'd wait until my husband slept and then sit up all night on the internet, ordering things and booking holidays we could never have taken with a tiny baby. I was very argumentative with friends or family who questioned my beliefs, I felt hugely frustrated that they couldn't see things the way I could and couldn't understand why they wanted to cause me distress by questioning things I said. I've since been told that as I'm fairly financially savvy in "real life" my arguments sometimes made a lot of sense. Some friends even began to wonder if perhaps I was actually still sane and had just done some very clever sums about our finances! Of course I'd actually done some very wrong sums, which would ultimately leave us with about three thousand pounds of debts to repay. So, what was happening to my baby boy at this time? Well, I was looking after his daily physical needs – nappy changes, baths, feeds, breast-feeding even slightly improved and I introduced some bottles too. But I wasn't "with him" emotionally, and much of the breast-feeding was done with him perched on my lap whilst I made lists or surfed the web for things to buy. Instead of being focused on getting to know him and spending quality time to bond I was treating him as a set of chores that needed doing, that were interrupting all the other irrelevant planning and spending activities that were occupying my mind. All that manic-ness came to an end the day that a team of professionals knocked on my front door to assess me for sectioning under the mental health act. In the background, largely un-noticed by me, my husband and family had been trying to get help. What I haven't mentioned until now is that I'm a mental health professional myself. So when that team knocked on the door I recognised some of them and for one mad moment I thought they'd just called socially to visit me and my new baby! But as the assessment commenced I gained a panicked insight into the situation I was finding myself in. Frankly I was terrified, and I gave serious consideration to trying to leg it over our garden fence. Instead I managed to resurrect from my addled brain enough professional knowledge of the mental health act to say the right things to stop them sectioning me, and they agreed to me receiving treatment and support in my own home. So on that day I got heavily sedated by medication, and my recovery, of sorts, began. What I didn't understand then, but know now, is that I was suffering with post-partum psychosis, a rare mental illness that only affects approx one in 500 new mums."

Tracey went on to explain how she regained her mental health in her next blog post:

"Post-partum Psychosis – the long and winding road to recovery

It's taken me a while to get onto writing this second post about my ongoing journey through post-partum psychosis. I think that's partly because the recovery phase was the most painful for me. In those early weeks my uncontrollable emotions were projected outwards as mania, which was highly alarming to those around me but relatively joyful for me as I lost my grip on reality, worried about nothing and believed lots of exciting things were possible. The following months were the polar opposite, as once the medication had brought me down from the high my thoughts and emotions became increasingly inward facing and desperately negative. I lost myself in feelings of shame about how I'd failed my baby and my family, guilt about getting us into debt and a sense of hopelessness that I'd ever be able to regain a normal life, return to my career and be a good mum. Most of all I internalised the full impact of the stigma of being diagnosed with a mental illness, which had a hugely detrimental impact on my recovery because it stopped me being honest with myself and others about my continuing distress...

The sedating medication I was initially prescribed did make me sleep, almost solidly for three days in fact. No consideration had been given to breast-feeding, so I had to abruptly give that up once I took my first dose. That may have been the right decision given the state I was in, but I've since learnt that stopping breast-feeding abruptly can be detrimental to mental health. Anyway, I continued to take medication for four weeks, which gradually calmed the mania. During this period I had frequent visits from midwives, health visitors and mental health professionals. My husband had to take time off work as I wasn't allowed to be alone with my baby, and friends and family rallied around to help. That is, those we chose to be honest with helped, but we hid the reality from many others. I can't really understand now why we did that, but I suspect that stigma played a big part. In those early weeks there were some discussions about admitting me to a mother and baby unit (MBU), but we didn't take that option, partly because it was too far away for my husband to visit easily, and also because the idea terrified me. What was I afraid of? Yet again, I think it was primarily the stigma.

Looking back now I sometimes regret not taking up the MBU bed as I can see that intensive specialist support may have enabled a more complete recovery and better bonding with my baby, and I think it would have been really helpful to meet other women in the same situation.

Instead of being admitted I stayed home with a desperate desire to put it all behind me as soon as possible, go back to "normal" and cope like other mums did. The medication I was on prevented me from waking for night feeds, so when I was recovered enough for my husband to return to work I weaned myself off it, so I could take full responsibility for my baby. Within two months I managed to convince myself and my care team that I was well and I got myself discharged from their care. It was such a relief to believe I'd recovered, and that I no longer wore that label of having a mental illness. Retrospectively I want to slap myself for letting internalised stigma prevent me from seeking, and holding on to, as much specialist support as I could, and for not being honest about the anxiety and depression symptoms I was now experiencing. I truly hope that the societal shifts we now see with the anti stigma work of Time to Change and others will, over time, lead to more people being more honest about how they are really feeling. Oh, and by the way, I absolutely do not recommend stopping medication without medical advice and supervision. It was very foolish, and could have had terrible consequences.

Instead of being honest I tried to ignore and hide my continued unease, and carry on with the daily activities of caring for a baby. I coped reasonably well despite the distressing and negative thoughts that were invading my mind, and I was able to join a post-natal group set up by local health visitors for new mums. I count myself extremely lucky for that, as that group of mums have become lifelong friends, and our growing families have shared memorable times together for over ten years now, starting as weekly meet ups, and developing into regular outings, camping trips and many a boozy girls night. It's hard to imagine now that it took me six months to tell those lovely ladies that I was "different" as I was suffering from post-natal mental illness. They probably still don't realise that our early times together were often painful for me as I felt so ashamed and inadequate, whilst they all seemed to be coping like "proper" mums should. I believe that if those early group sessions with the health visitors had included information about post-natal mental health issues it would have been easier to be honest with those other mums, and to ask for the type of support and reassurance I really needed.

Eventually, after a few months of outwardly coping but being in secret emotional turmoil I could no longer contain it, and I broke down in tears during what was supposed to be a fun cinema outing with my husband. I finally admitted that I wasn't really coping and needed more help, and I went back under the care of the community mental health team, on a new medication regime and having regular visits. The medication took many weeks to properly lift my mood, so I continued to experience very negative thoughts and to worry constantly. Some of those thoughts are too painful to share, but I'll just say that I sit here today greatly relieved that I didn't act on them. I didn't always find the support from well meaning professionals helpful, as I wasn't given hope that I could fully recover, and the underlying issues weren't really addressed. Thankfully in the ten years since then mental health services have become much better at focusing on recovery and instilling hope.

What undoubtedly helped me hugely during that period was when I finally got to see a specialist perinatal mental health team, who explained my diagnosis and told me that most women with post-partum psychosis do fully recover, learn to love being a mum, and regain fulfilling lives. And over time my own experience has showed that to be true. There were certainly many emotional struggles for many more months, and it's taken many years to let go of the guilt and shame, and to feel like a "good enough" mum, but I was able to start a gradual return to work when my baby was nine months old, and I've successfully continued to develop my career in mental health, juggling that with the joy of bringing up my incredible little boy.

And here's the other great thing – I went on to have a beautiful daughter too! ... the perinatal mental health team supported me to enable that to happen, despite the fact that there is a 50:50 chance of post-partum psychosis recurring in women who have had it before."

23

The effect on men

The women who shared their stories with me often mentioned their partners – the role they played, and the support they gave. But I wanted to find out more about how PND affected them. Rightly, the focus tends to be on the sufferer, who does have to take priority. But it's important not to exclude partners in any consideration of perinatal mental illness. They play – or can play – such a huge role in helping women recover from PND, and the experience can obviously have a big impact on them too. And there is a growing understanding that fathers are at risk of depression in the post-natal period too.

Sam's story

Sam is 37, and though he now lives abroad he and his wife had their two children while living in the UK. Like the majority of dads, he took the standard two weeks paternity leave from his job when each of his children was born. Looking back on what he thought fatherhood would be like, he says, "my expectations were that it would be something I would love in the long term, but I was apprehensive about the early days and how we would be able to look after a baby." His concerns were borne out when his first child was born: "I was shocked by the relentlessness... it is a 24 hour day, 365 days a year job, you never get a break." Both he and his wife had been very keen to have children, and he had felt confident that his wife would adapt well to motherhood.

For Sam and his partner, they sound unsupported from the point they were back at home, after the birth. Disappointed by their health visitors – who he thinks put them in the "all right, can cope" category, and basically left them alone – they struggled to access help for problems like breast-feeding. They did not have family close to home, and he comments that, in hindsight, his wife regrets not asking for more help from her mother. The couple had taken part in antenatal classes with the NCT, and he reflects that perhaps he could have done with more preparation for the post-birth period – although he acknowledges that "no amount of talking or classes is really going to prepare you." So with little support from extended family or in the community, Sam was very much the primary supporter, which he says he would not have wanted any other way. "We have a close and supportive marriage in all areas and I would have been upset if I wasn't the primary source of support." The birth of their first child he describes as "brutal (the pain and the blood)". As first labours go, 13 hours was not too terrible, but they had a familiar problem in convincing the midwives they dealt with that his wife was in established labour. As a pre-eclampsia sufferer myself, I was interested to hear that Sam's wife had it with both children. In a similar first labour to my own, she had actually gone into natural labour before being given Syntocinon during induction, but the midwives were sceptical that she could be in 'real' labour without the drug.

Both babies were born at 38 weeks because of the pre-eclampsia. This early arrival meant that the couple felt unprepared first time around, having only just moved house and not even had time to build their crib. Amid the chaos, Sam was sent home at 11pm and then summoned back in at 1.30am. But, he says, "I was very proud of my wife throughout the whole process and thankfully there were no major problems for either mother or baby." Second time around was "very different", partly because his wife had an epidural. The labour was quicker, and the couple felt more prepared. "The whole experience was much calmer and there was only a single midwife there most of the time." I asked Sam if he bonded with his first child straightaway, and he queried what I meant by that. That made me realise that perhaps it's a question just mothers tend to get – we definitely (or perhaps it's just those with PND) get very used to GPs, Health Visitors and therapists saying "and how is bonding?" He says he remembers wondering how they would cope after their first child's birth, rather than instantly feeling pride or happiness. But, "I thought she was wonderful and I was very proud, but it was very hard work. I have a much stronger bond with my children now than when they were babies." He comments that his partner revealed later that she felt she hadn't bonded with their first child early on. The first few weeks were very tough: the baby screamed a lot. "I know that all babies cry, but our first child seemed to do it more than other babies." They introduced a dummy and this improved matters – their daughter began to sleep well at night. But she continued to scream during the day: "I know my wife used to count the minutes until I came home." From a practical point of view this meant no respite for whichever parent was looking after the baby: she could not be put down, so basic tasks like taking a shower or making lunch were impossible. "Holding her didn't stop the screaming but at least you felt you were doing something. During the worst times, my wife and I used to do 20 minute shifts with our first child and then swap."

About two or three months in, Sam realised that his wife was depressed. "I didn't know what to do or where to seek help. Part of the problem was that I think my wife wouldn't admit it to herself. She's always been a coper and has a horror of medication for depression (she's been prescribed it during a couple of periods outside of the PND period and has never taken it)." He himself did not have anyone he could confide in – he says his wife would rather have died than let him speak to his mother. Despite all this, he does not himself think he suffered from depression.

The couple did not consult their doctor or any other professional for help. He says this was because his wife "didn't want to admit to herself that she was depressed". She was never asked by a health visitor about her mental health.

Compounding this, or perhaps one of the causes of it, both babies suffered from reflux in the early months. Their first baby was a very "sicky" baby – fed well but "posseted" a lot. This instantly reminded me of how we had to buy a throw for our sofa when Joe was a baby because it became irreparably stained by all the baby sick… he now thinks that all the screaming may have been because she was in pain.

Their second child had serious problems feeding and, as a result, did not grow. "We regularly spent eight hours of the day with a bottle in her mouth trying to get her to take the milk (she absolutely refused to breast-feed after three months of age)." Unlike her older sister, this baby did not scream or seem to be in pain – but obviously the fact she was not growing was a cause of great anxiety to her parents. As with many couples, the advent of their second child brought in new difficulties, as the couple tried to juggle the two. Sam says the first 18 months of her life were hard, given the feeding difficulties. In that first year or so, he feels they had not time to devote to their older child, and she would spend a lot of time in front of the TV.

Despite the setbacks, and the couple not having much external support, he says that having a family brought them closer together, rather than driving a wedge between them as some couples have experienced. He enjoyed making new friends after having his child, and says he was "always proud to show off my child. I also enjoyed being a hands-on dad – I liked to think I was a bit different (and a bit better) than the others!" He also says he feels they have definitely moved past the difficult starts they had. "Our children are an absolute delight (and become more so every day)." But despite this, they remain realistic because of their experience. "We always wanted three, but the experience of the early months and years is one of the reasons we will probably not have any more. We are scared it will happen again."

Mark's story

Mark Williams experience of post- natal depression both as a partner looking on, and experiencing it himself as a father, made such an impression that he's set up two support groups: Fathers Reaching Out and Dads Matter UK. The first thing he says is that it is very hard to get men to speak up, and he's talking from experience – he was that man. Fathers Reaching Out was primarily set up to support dads whose partners are suffering from PND, which was the situation Mark found himself in after his son was born in 2004. Following a traumatic birth by emergency C-section, his wife developed severe PND. She was so badly affected that Mark gave up his job so he could support her at home.

"When I started [campaigning about PND and dads] four or five years ago, I was laughed at" he remarks. He thinks that in that time there has already been a shift towards more awareness and understanding – a shift that arguably he has been partly behind, as he has written, spoken and campaigned about PND in both fathers and mothers extensively. He thinks that often fathers looking after a partner with PND don't want to tell their partner that they themselves are feeling low, out of protectiveness and concern that it might exacerbate the mother's condition. So instead, they often try to hide how they are feeling. When Mark 's son was born he was 30, and he says neither he or his wife had experienced mental illness before then. He himself was traumatised by the birth, and describes the doctors coming in to talk to him, with "no expression" on their faces – he suffered a panic attack, fearing for his wife and son's lives. Now, he says he could never contemplate going through that again, and the couple have changed their original plans to have two children.

They were fortunate, he says, to have a very good Community Psychiatric Nurse who later went on to specialise in perinatal mental health. But having been self-employed, and now not in work so that he could help his wife, the family faced serious money worries. He mentions several times that although his wife was very ill, her bonding was never affected: it was more that she battled with a perception of herself as a bad mother. He remembers this time as feeling like "there was no end in sight... I isolated myself."

He points to the problem of stigma around mental health, and PND in particular, being an obstacle to speaking out. His mother-in-law came to stay with the family to help them. In hindsight, he can clearly see he himself was depressed. "I was getting thoughts, my personality was changing. My mates asked what the matter was?" And he turned to drinking as a way to cope. He remembers having suicidal thoughts, and his mind racing. This period – when their baby was six to eight months old – stands out as a crisis point for Mark. But it wasn't until 2011 – seven years after his son was born – that he started to realise what had happened to him. He went through a series of traumatic events – family bereavements – which led to a breakdown. All his issues resurfaced, and he says his body basically shut down. He sought help from his GP, was given medication – citalopram – and put on the waiting list for counselling which he notes he has still never had. Fortunately he was able to pay for private counselling for alcohol dependency, along with eight CBT sessions. Around this time, having headed to the gym on the basis that exercise could help his mood, he found himself chatting to a man sitting alongside him lifting weights. Within ten minutes the pair had realised they had much in common: the man's wife had also had PND, and he himself was suffering from depression – just like Mark. It was an epiphany for Mark, who realised firstly that he was not alone, and secondly that talking side by side was a way in which men could open up to each other – rather than face to face. "I told him more in ten minutes than I had told my best mates". That realisation, coupled with the discovery when he searched online that there was really no support out there for fathers like him, led to him setting up Fathers Reaching Out.

It was only with his breakdown in 2011 that Mark realised some of his feelings could be traced back to 2004, when his son was born. He said he knew "if I didn't get help, the suicidal thoughts would come back". He retrained as a mental health advocate, and along with his wife does a lot of voluntary work in the community with young people. His outlook is that his experience has changed his view of life. He has less money now, but he loves what he is doing. Most recently he has given up his job as a mental health advocate so that he can focus on campaigning for perinatal mental health awareness full time.

As well as taking citalopram, he says CBT and mindfulness were crucial to recovery. He looks back and thinks it all started with the birth itself. He felt anxious: "who was this stranger coming into my life, what had he done to my wife?" He also showed OCD traits in the weeks after the birth, checking on the baby and his wife constantly.

Mark hits on a massive change which fatherhood brings: the different role. That's particularly true in cases where the mother has PND. Suddenly he was in "a caring role", and his wife was reacting differently to him. "We used to bounce off each other". He became so frustrated he punched the sofa and broke his hand, which he comments made changing nappies quite difficult...

And, on top of this, he talks about the problems men have opening up to each other. But in the meantime, if, for instance, the birth has been traumatic, anything can trigger off a feeling of anxiety: a smell, seeing a baby in the street, meeting a pregnant woman.

When their son was a baby, Mark and his wife had just moved into a new home. Their lifestyle changed completely, as many new parents discover; suddenly they were not going out any more. But on top of that, of course, both were struggling with depression, even though Mark did not know it at the time. They moved to a different house, for a new start.

Mark offers an insight into the mind of a father whose partner has PND, saying that, having never experienced mental illness before, he was asking himself, "how could she be depressed? We have everything." He gave her the credit card and urged her to go shopping and make herself happy. He now knows that it doesn't work that way, of course.

Now, he is very much at the centre of perinatal mental health campaigning. He cites the NCT's report on depression in dads, which suggests that more than one in three new dads are concerned about their mental health.[9] But he feels there is much, much more to do. He would like to see more research into suicide rates of new fathers, for instance. And he talks about the teenage fathers he has met through his work in the mental health services. Many of them just simply don't know about issues like depression, or how their partner might change after motherhood. He comes back again to that idea of men talking side by side. "If the father is well, there's an increased chance the mum will get better," he says.

---

9 NCT "Dads in distress: Many new fathers are worried about their mental health" 18 June 2015

24

Opening up

Blogger Susan DeBake's story

Susan DeBake writes a blog – Life in Full Bloom – which details her experience of PND (or post-partum depression as it's known in the US, where she is from). Interestingly her experience actually began before the birth, as she details in her blog. This post is from when she opened up for the first time about her depression:

"How I knew it was more than 'just hormones' – PART TWO
7 Replies

In my previous post, I talked about the reason why it is so dangerously easy for women suffering from post-partum (or prenatal) depression to think, "Oh, it's just the hormones." Because, after all, we've been saying and hearing that our entire lives.

I want to preface this post by saying this: HINDSIGHT IS 20/20. And that really sucks, huh?!? No fair! If only we had clarity and common sense and objectiveness DURING our trials instead of AFTER! But alas, it is what it is, and I'm grateful that now I'm looking at things in hindsight and not in the depths of it.

When I was seven months pregnant with my second baby (my adorably charming son, Anders, now 21 months old), my husband and I went on a much-needed date. While we were waiting for our food to arrive, my husband looked me in the eye, and said, "How ARE you?" And to thank him for such a kind question, I started sobbing. You guys, I don't mean like, oh, sniff, a tear! But, GUSH, swollen nose, red eyes, snot and drool. NOT pretty. Poor AJ. He was flabbergasted.

I told him, "I'm just so hormonal… " And then the moment came. I knew I needed to TALK to him, to tell him that, maybe, just maybe? it was MORE than "just hormones" and that, maybe? I was actually depressed. I told him we'd talk when we got home, that P.F. Chang's other customers didn't deserve to see or hear what I had to say. :-) And when we got home, I talked. And cried.

This was a pivotal moment for me; it was the first time I'd said the word "depressed" to my husband. I told him how I'd been feeling that everything was pointless and that I just couldn't get excited about things anymore. I told him I felt like I was walking around outside of myself, watching me interact but not truly being present. I knew he didn't fully understand; how could he? But he listened and was supportive. And life continued.

I gave birth to Anders on April 5, 2012. He was 8lb 10oz (2 oz shy of his big sister!) and we were so excited. My healthy, strong baby boy was delivered after 3 pushes and being in the hospital for 2 hours. Talk about easy!

But then I tried to breast-feed. And all of my horrible

memories of trying to feed my daughter came flooding back. Even our lactation consultant was the same one we had with her!! And Anders had the same exact issue as his sister: he literally could not open his mouth wide enough to feed properly. So we went home.

Anders was a perfect little champ (except in the feeding area) for the next four weeks. He was a very typical baby, waking every three hrs or so, and otherwise just sleeping all day. To be honest, I don't really remember too much of those first five weeks. **This is, in hindsight, the first big symptom of my post-partum depression: I was not fully present in my surroundings.** It was a complete fog. I was going through the motions.

But I do remember when we first started noticing his acid reflux (how can one forget your child SHRIEKING in pain?!?) and the many, many doctor visits and the trial and error tests of formulas and prescription medicines and refusal to eat and his loss of weight and general discomfort ALL DAY AND NIGHT LONG. His doctor asked me, "How are you doing?" and I said, "It's been a long month" and I distinctly remember thinking, "Don't cry, don't cry, you're just tired. It's just the hormones." He was about six weeks old at this point.

I had my six week check-up with my OB. I was still sore (I had 3rd degree perineal tearing) but was healing fine. She said, "Any symptoms of depression?" and I said, "Oh, you know, the usual hormonal stuff... "

What I didn't tell these doctors (kind, caring, professional women who have known me for years, by the way) was that every time I tried to get Anders to fall asleep and he didn't (which was quite often) **I would be so overcome with ANGER and RAGE** that I would literally leave him, crying, in his swing, while I fell to the floor shaking and sobbing.

What I didn't tell them was that when I attended any sort of social function, **I felt that my speech was stuttered.** That I literally couldn't form a complete sentence and say it properly.

What I didn't tell them was that during the night, during those precious few hours **when my son was actually asleep, I was wide awake, my mind restless and unrelenting.**

I didn't tell them that in general, **I just didn't care**. Don't get me wrong; I loved my children desperately, and, thank the Lord, I never once felt that I was going to harm anyone, even myself. But, when I wasn't overcome with anger, **I had an extreme apathy for everything**. My daughter's laugh on the swing didn't make me smile. Her interactions with her baby brother made me feel, if anything, a desperate hopelessness that I would never be the mother they really needed.

I didn't tell anyone that **all day, every day, I felt like a failure**.

One of my darkest moments came when Anders was about eight weeks old. As usual, I was trying to get him to sleep ANYWHERE BUT IN MY ARMS and was failing. My entire being filled with an inexplicable anger. I put him in the swing and sank to the floor, sobbing tears that were desperately uncontrollable. My mind was completely blank yet so out of control that literally the only thing I could think of to pray was the name of Jesus. I said it out loud: "Jesus", over and over and over again until I finally calmed down. And then I prayed, "Please, please, please, don't let my children be affected by this. *Protect them from this, from me.*"

It was that prayer that made me realise that maybe I needed help. The fact that one day, my children might say, "yeah, my mom was depressed a lot" scared the daylights out of me. I needed to get help, even if just to protect my children from the effects of living with someone with unmanaged depression.

My best friend visited from New Hampshire the next week. She is like a sister to me, and I've always been able to be completely honest with her. Talking about how I was feeling was such a relief. I told her what I was experiencing, and she saw it firsthand. She did not judge me, nor did she say, "oh, it's probably just the hormones." She was able to look at my situation objectively and simply said, "You need to get help. You need to call your doctor." What a wise, beautiful woman she is.

I finally saw my doctor about four weeks later. FOUR WEEKS!! It truly is amazing that, in the midst of feeling so out of control, the last thing I wanted to do was to talk to my doctor about it. As I've mentioned before, admitting you struggle with depression is the hardest step."

What I really enjoy about this blog is the fact that Susan concentrates on recovery, rather than just chronicling her depression (which in itself would be a valid blog, but it's helpful to see how other people manage their depression on a practical level.). In a post entitled "My Battle Plan: 7 ways I'm fighting depression" she sets out the artillery she has lined up for the fight. She is clear that it's a multi-layered approach, and that no one element on its own would suffice. Number 1 on the list is "I am on an anti-depressant." She is very up-front about this, saying that when her son was ten weeks old, she felt overcome by the "dark, all-consuming and sometimes frantic world", and could barely form a sentence. Her doctor prescribed Sertraline, which initially Susan was unsure about taking. She wondered if taking it would mean she was "now certifiably crazy". She is a committed Christian, and I suspect that for those who have a strong faith, while that can undoubtedly be an enormous source of strength in the face of depression, it may also present dilemmas: should you take external help such as medication? And Susan writes that this was the case for her, she certainly worried that "if I took this medicine, I'd be turning my back on [God]." However, friends and family counselled her that she had a medical condition that should be treated as such. She is clear about Sertraline and how it works, the fact that it is not "a happy pill... But what it did do was pull the dark cloud back just enough for me to see my situation in a more objective way. I wasn't all of a sudden 'Happy! Yay! Isn't life grand!' But I stopped feeling overwhelmed with anger. I stopped sobbing for hours. I started noticing when my daughter laughed and my son smiled. I started to see clearly for the first time in months, and I could finally breathe." I love the way Susan writes, with such a light touch but absolutely spot on about the highs and lows of life with PND.

Once the medication kicked in and allowed Susan "to come up for air", she started exercising regularly. She tries to go the gym four to five times a week, saying she notices the effect on her mood if she goes less often. She is fortunate to have some very supportive friends, and indeed a very supportive husband. She suggests that if you are suffering from PND and don't have friends who will properly check in on you – asking what they can do and how you are that day – perhaps it is worth finding a therapist so that you have someone to truly talk to.

Sleep, of course, is at the root or at least an exacerbating factor for so many of us with PND. And Susan is emphatic that getting enough sleep is crucial. She tries to take naps when she can during the day. Just like her awareness that missing a few gym sessions starts to have an effect on her mood, she comments, "If I go too long with poor sleep, I really notice my mood gets terrible. This happens to anyone! And it can

be especially dangerous for someone battling depression."
As well as the naps, she enlists her husband's help when she
is struggling with bad nights. He steps up and helps and she
puts the earplugs in. The couple prioritise time away from
the children – booking babysitters and having nights out –
and Susan organises time for herself too. She's also mindful
of her diet and the effect that can have on mental health.

Her disclaimer makes me laugh:

Disclaimer:

I am not a medical professional, nor do I play one on TV.
The comments and opinions expressed in these articles are
merely comments and opinions. Please seek professional
medical advice before making any changes to the diet,
exercise, or medication of yourself or your children.

25

The beginning of the end

When my son was around two, my mum asked me if I would write about my experience of post-natal depression for her church magazine. I agreed, and the short piece I wrote is what grew into this book. There was another contributor, whose words I found so beautifully put and articulate, they have stayed with me. She has kindly agreed to share them here.

C's story

"When my daughter was born they took her away into special care and I was sure there was something terribly wrong with her. Actually, as it turned out, she was only there for ten minutes, and it was me that was taken to theatre to stop me from losing dangerous amounts of blood. During the hour that I was away, my husband held our baby daughter and rocked her, and cuddled her and learned about her. He probably had more contact immediately than most fathers ever get the chance to have. When I got back, he was able to tell me things about her that I didn't know - like she sucked her tongue the whole time and it was just her being hungry.

And then afterwards, it seemed a lifetime but it can only have been perhaps a week - because a week is a lifetime when you have a new baby, and simultaneously no time at all - I watched her throwing shapes in her Moses basket, my little daughter raving to the great god of wind. And it is all wind in the first months, wind and confusion. And I remember great aching waves of emotion, joy and terror and excitement and hysteria, and the clear sense that we absolutely must get on with the business of having another one as soon as possible. And this sense of confidence and joy lasting perhaps a month, perhaps as long as six weeks, before my brain chemicals threw me a curve ball and I started to slide hopelessly into a state of total paranoia and anxiousness and control-freakery that even I could recognise was wildly irrational and exhausting and mad.

I was still in it in May when she was three months old. We had a freak hailstorm. Hailstones as big as smarties, bouncing off the attic windows, setting off car alarms, decimating our courgette plants. There was so much hail forcing its way down drainpipes and backing up in drains that a section of downpipe exploded in a geyser of icy water. And this felt like my mind. Sheer nervous energy, relentless pressure, unimaginable boredom and hormonal overload combining to push my mental capacity until it fractured and I shook and screamed and sobbed and hated myself and my life and my husband and sometimes even my baby: but always when she was asleep. Only when she was asleep. Because when she is awake she must only have sane, smiling Mummy.

So I asked the doctor for pills, and read the literature about anti-depressants and breast-feeding, and tried to find a way to make a rational decision - this with my brain chemistry wearing its shoes on the wrong feet. And my mind circled the question with increasing intensity: should I stop breast-feeding? Can I introduce formula at four months? The feeding police tell me I should carry on breast-feeding exclusively until six months... but my mother introduced solids at eight weeks and we were all fine? If I breast-feed on anti-depressants, will they affect the baby? If I take old style anti-depressants they seem to be safer for breast-feeding, but they have nasty side-effects, including weight gain which I can guarantee will trigger depression all of its own.

So we bring on the bottle. We move to half and half feeding. And every breastfeed I don't give feels like a betrayal and every bottle feed I do give feels like a blessed relief. I still don't take the pills because there is always something I might need to breast-feed her through: her vaccinations, the possibility of chickenpox, the disruption of going to nursery. And I see that this will never end, no matter how old she is and whether she is weaned, or walking or twenty or having babies of her own I will always want to give her something of myself to make her feel better, and it will never be enough because she will need her own good mental health. And for me to teach her how to develop her mental health, I must have mine."

When I left therapy, when my second son was about a year old, my GP was sent a letter from my therapist:

"... Ms Hargreave attended a course of individual Cognitive Behaviour Therapy (CBT) and we had our final follow-up session on 9th September 2012...

Ms Hargreave made very good progress towards her goals and committed to therapy throughout the sessions. At the start of treatment, Ms Hargreave scored 11 on the PHQ-9 and nine on the GAD-7 which indicated moderate depression and mild anxiety. At the end of treatment Ms Hargreave scored two on the PHQ-9 and one on the GAD-7 which indicated minimal depression and anxiety.

Ms Hargreave has been encouraged to continue to apply all that she has learnt in therapy to new situations and no further therapy is indicated at present… "

The letters and grades the therapist mentions refer to the standard questionnaires I had to fill in every week before my sessions. You can tell from the scores my therapist reports that I had made clear progress (though obviously therapy is measured by more than just numbers). When nearing the end of therapy, I was encouraged to develop my own "blueprint", a map of what my goals were, a reminder of what my particular triggers were and suggestions for how to combat my own bêtes noirs. When I read this letter, I realised that, despite not feeling it every day, things had definitely changed. I sought out an old email from when I first went on anti-depressants. I had written to a friend:

"… he's really really grizzly at the moment, no idea why. I'm much the same really, except with the added complication of a possible infection where my stitches were… ugh! and ow! Just feel as though I'm making no progress at all, everything still feels v bleak and impossible. Hopefully the drugs will kick in soon. And I will hopefully get referred to someone who can help me as well. I'm just so sick of feeling like this, just seem to spend hours crying and feeling incapable, and nothing anyone says seems to help. I think Ben is considering taking some leave so he can be with me more but that is finite - and quite precious time - so not sure really."

And the day after, in response to a very supportive and caring message she sent me:

"… really does help to get a message like this. I saw doc yesterday so have antibiotics for stitches. Think Joe has a cold.

I think it's just hard to see the bigger picture at the moment - Ben thinks things are vastly improved but I can't really see it at the moment, and still feel incapable of going out and about very much with him. I had a meltdown at 7am this morning when it was time for a feed and I'd only had three hours sleep all night - Ben ended up sending me back to bed while he did the feed. Think you are right about getting some rest!

… haven't sorted out any counselling or support groups yet. My GP has referred me to a specialist counsellor but says it's likely to be a long wait… Think you're right about the groups - it's just a bit of a step to actually call someone I don't know. One of the links you sent me the other day was about cognitive behavioural therapy which sounded interesting. I think as well as the meds it's definitely a case of trying to change some of the mindset that this is impossible and will never get any easier.

… better go, we're getting a taxi up to Great Ormond Street in a bit so need to get Joe ready. Am meeting Ben there which is itself a big step, going on my own, even if it is in the comfort of a taxi!"

Then, as now, it was hard to gain perspective, and to step outside of myself and properly appreciate the recovery which was underway. And I think those messages emphasise what other women have said about taking anti-depressants. There clearly wasn't an identifiable moment when things got better. But they helped in a gradual way. So much so that when I first decided to come off Sertraline, about a year after Joe was born, I was very anxious about how I would cope without them. I wanted to come off them because I believed (wrongly) that I had to if I wanted to become pregnant again. By odd coincidence, I had discovered not long after I started Sertraline that my aunt, a pharmaceutical consultant who used to work at Pfizer, had been involved in the latter stages of the development of Sertraline. When Joe was about a year old, I emailed her for advice:

"… Also wanted to ask your advice about coming off Sertraline. I'm going to my GP of course about it but I thought I'd ask you too. I'm on 50mg, once a day. I've been on it for a year and would like to come off (I realise this has to be gradual) partly to see how I do without it and partly as we want to start thinking about another baby this year… I admit I'm quite nervous both about withdrawal symptoms and how I'll fare off the medication, but I'm going to ask about CBT counselling on the NHS as I'd like to try that if I can. I'm also very very nervous about getting post-natal depression again (this is all assuming I can get pregnant of course!). I have heard that sometimes you can take Sertraline pre-emptively in cases like this, even in your last month of pregnancy - so will ask the doctor. It would preclude breast-feeding but I would rather be mentally well. I also need to ask about pre-eclampsia but suspect that much like the PND they won't be able to predict whether I'll get it again or not."

My aunt was very supportive throughout, and her reply was no exception. She gave me practical advice on cutting down Sertraline very gradually (though of course I did also consult my own GP on this, who concurred with my aunt's suggestions). My aunt also said this, which I found intriguing:

"… There's no reason why you should have PND again after another baby - Mummy had it severely after your dad was born and was fine after [my uncle]. In the unlikely event that you did, you know the symptoms and could go back on the Sertraline."

I knew my own mother had *not* suffered from PND, but now it turned out my paternal grandmother had – although

I suspect it wasn't recognised as such at the time. I had forgotten all about this until I began writing this book, so I went back to ask my aunt if she could remember anything else. What she told me was fascinating. She said that, while living in India and after having had my father, my grandmother suffered from "what was described as puerperal psychosis, but perhaps it was what would now be classified as PND." Apparently she was already ill by the time she was in labour with my father, because she had insisted on delivering him on a chair in the waiting room at the hospital, refusing to be admitted to the maternity ward. This was followed by three months in hospital, during which time my grandmother's elder two children were housed in a convent. Her eldest (my uncle) could remember my grandmother turning her face to the wall when her children visited her in hospital. And my aunt recalls that my grandmother insisted my father had been one of twins, and accused the hospital staff of stealing the other baby. My aunt, then two years old, when reunited with her mother clung to a nun's skirts asking, "who is that lady?" and feels that the three month separation possibly affected their bonding. My grandfather was a Police Superintendent and very busy with his work in another part of the country. My aunt suspects the resulting strain on him affected his relationship with my own father, who was always labelled a difficult child. Meanwhile my grandmother was a long way away from home, and her own mother had died before her second child was born. My aunt says, "There is a photo of me sitting on Mummy's knee which I think may have been taken just after she came out of hospital. She certainly doesn't look well."

I was quite fixated on the need to come off anti-depressants first time around, and I repeated the way I had done this when Ted was about a year old. But it was not the right time, and a few months later I was in a doctor's office sobbing hysterically and saying through the tears, "I think maybe it was a bit too soon..?" When Joe was little and he suddenly stopped sleeping through at about nine months, I realised something quite important about parenting. There are no absolutes. You (or your child) master something, and then it all changes. They sleep, they don't. They eat, suddenly they don't. Nothing stands still. And in the same way, I've come to realise that mental wellbeing is the same. You don't "feel better" and necessarily keep feeling better. Just like raising children, it's all about good days and bad days.

Epilogue

We take a battering from PND. It is certainly the hardest thing I have gone through. But on the other hand... there is Joe. He's my first-born, he's grown into a little boy with multiple layers, he's a mass of contradictions and he's brilliant. He's madcap but he worries about the human race and why everyone has to die. He loves toilet humour but he thinks that different beliefs can be accommodated because whatever you believe in, will come true, so if you believe in reincarnation you could come back as something else. He tells me he loves me many, many times a day. His memory stretches back to before his second birthday, and continually amazes me; it surpasses that of his approaching middle-aged mum. I am grateful though that it doesn't stretch back further: I don't want him ever doubting for one minute that he is loved. Joe is learning how to tell jokes, and he hasn't quite got the hang of it, so knock knock might turn into a fascinating Skylanders fact delivered at high volume. He is a boy who learnt how to sing Three Little Birds and loves it, following his granny into an unlikely Bob Marley appreciation. He's a boy who loves the Wizard of Oz but hates Frozen.

He's bright, he's highly strung, he's funny, and he's ours. We fight like cat and dog and it's probably because we are very alike. We love each other passionately, and he makes me laugh as much as my brother does, which means a lot, more than almost anyone else. I treasure his most recent school picture, not because it is the best, but because I know the backstory which led to the pursed lips, carefully covering up a dangling loose tooth; he declared "Ugerly". He asks me on the way to school, "what happened when I was born?" as if he knows what I'm writing about in this book. I tell him a bit, and he says, "and did you cry?"" Yes," I say. "The midwife told me, 'your baby has black hair' and I cried so much, the anaesthetist asked if I was in pain. 'No,' I told him, 'I'm just emotional.'" I explained to Joe that this meant I was crying happy tears. He knew what that meant because a teacher did that when the children sang Happy Birthday to her. I have started to explain to him that sometimes mummies don't feel so well after their babies are born, and they might feel quite unhappy: but that doesn't mean they don't love their child, and that I was like that – but I got better.

Joe is enormous tantrums, terrifying rage, tears-flying drama. He is the introvert's extrovert child, and I have been amused over the years by how many social situations I've ended up in which would never have occurred without his craving for other people, for contact, for conversation. He gets sentimental at bedtime, never more so than the night he said to me, "Mummy… when I was little, before I was even born, I wished for a mummy with brown eyes, brown hair, glasses, a golden bag and a golden phone… and that is exactly what I got." I am not overly sentimental, but I was touched by this insight into his world, and his view of me. And I do have all those things. But I also have him.

And then, there is Ted. Ted is corkscrew curls, which he never lets me comb. Ted is sticky hands clasped round my neck, setting off chronic back pain because I can't say no to carrying him. Ted is the most cherubic sleeping child I've ever seen (he took two years to learn how to sleep, so it's lucky that, now he does, he does it beautifully). Ted is a constant babble, and he lives in "Ted's house" which is in "Ted's world", he sleeps in "Ted's bed". When we get near Joe's school, he says we are in "Joe's world". I talk to him about his "blue, blue eyes" and so that's how he prefaces any mention of eyes. He lies prostrate on the bedroom floor on the mornings it's not my turn to get up. An ill-fated stint in nursery ended when a staff member said, "he doesn't really seem to concentrate on what we ask him to do," and that's because he is immersed in what he's doing, and that is fine. And by fine, I don't mean fine (not fine). I really mean it is ok. During a recent trip to A&E he in turn charmed everyone ("That's daddy!" "I'm all better!") and broke our hearts ("I don't *want* to be brave"… I do wonder what we are doing to our children with all our exhortations that they be brave? It's like Warhorse at the doctors). He told me just tonight, "I love all of you", and of course I feel the same way about him.

Like everyone's children, mine can't really be summed up in a few words. I've noticed since having two that people tend to "look for the differences" – something you'll hear twin parents say. But actually the differences – and likenesses – are very subtle sometimes, and it is not usually a question of "the quiet one" and "the loud one". My two are so, so alike. And so very different. The luckiest thing of all is that for now they seem to love each other.

I never knew, back when the dark cloud obscured everything, that there would come a time when my kids would shriek "Mumeeeee!" with such delight it would be like closing my eyes on the beach and feeling the sun beat through them. Daily life is a grind, but loving them, and being loved by them, is the point.

Resources

During my experience of being a mother I have come across various outstanding organisations and resources which others may find useful. Throughout the writing of this book I have been pointed towards many more – more than I was able to do justice to in the context of this book. They include:

www.bluebellcare.org - Bristol-based post-natal care charity

www.bestbeginnings.org.uk - National charity which campaigns to improve the health of babies across the UK, and which has produced the award-winning Baby Buddy app.

www.maternalmentalhealthalliance.org.uk/ - Alliance of charities campaigning on improving perinatal mental health care in the UK, and creators of the everyonesbusiness.org.uk campaign

www.family-action.org.uk - National charity focused on families experiencing poverty, disadvantage or social isolation in England

www.reachingoutpmh.co.uk - Dads Matter UK/ Fathers Reaching Out

www.pandasfoundation.org.uk – Pre- and Post- Natal Depression advice and support

www.apni.org - Association for Post-Natal Illness

www.app-network.org - UK Post-partum Psychosis network

www.home-start.org.uk - Family support charity

www.tommys.org - Baby charity, provides excellent resources for pregnant women

www.thesmilegroup.org - The Smile Group, support group based in Cheshire, run by mothers who have experienced PND

www.mind.org.uk - Mind, the mental health charity, provides specific resources on PND.

www.helenabelgrave.co.uk - Dr Helena Belgrave, counselling psychologist

www.dulwichpsychologist.co.uk - Dr Christine Langhoff, clinical psychologist

Acknowledgements

My biggest debt is to all the mothers – and fathers – who have shared their stories here, with great courage and generosity. To protect their identities, names have been changed, but they know who they are, and I am very grateful to each of them. Thank you Tracey Robinson and Susan DeBake for kindly sharing extracts of their respective blogs here. I am also grateful to all my friends, family and colleagues who I have discussed PND with over the years, both in terms of my own experience and the issue generally – it's all led me to this point, and to this book, which I hope will be helpful to other families affected in the same way. Thank you to all of you who encouraged me to go ahead and write this book. And to Alice Solomons at Free Association Books, who gave me the opportunity to see it in print.

I have been very fortunate in the professionals in the field who have generously given me their time and access to their considerable expertise on perinatal mental health issues. It is always easier to focus on where we are lacking – and sadly, in perinatal mental health, there is still much that is lacking – but the professionals I have spoken to in the writing of this book tell a different story. It is heartening to hear of some of the outstanding work which is going on, and the success stories these people tell proves the value of their work. So Dr Helena Belgrave, Dr Rebecca Moore, Dr Christine Langhoff, Dr Tara George, Stacy Woodward, Sam Wilkinson, Dr Beckie Lang, Maria Bavetta, Ruth Jackson: thank you.